THE BLENDED FAMILY ACTIVITY BOOK FOR KIDS

the BLENDED FAMILY ACTIVITY BOOK for KIDS

FOR AGES 6-9

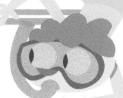

50 FUN ACTIVITIES TO HELP CHILDREN NAVIGATE CHANGE

April Eldemire, LMFT

Illustrations by Amir Abou-Roumié

ROCKRIDGE PRESS

For general information on our other products and services or to obtain technical support, please contact our Customer Care Department within the United States at (866) 744-2665, or outside the United States at (510) 253-0500.

Rockridge Press publishes its books in a variety of electronic and print formats. Some content that appears in print may not be available in electronic books, and vice versa.

Interior and Cover Designer: Heather Krakora
Art Producer: Melissa Malinowksy
Editor: Brian Sweeting
Production Editor: Ruth Sakata Corley
Production Manager: Jose Olivera

Illustration © 2021 Amir Abou-Roumié

Paperback ISBN: 978-1-63807-195-2
eBook ISBN: 978-1-63807-587-5
R0

TO MY SON OLIVER,
WHO HAS TAUGHT ME
HOW TO FORGIVE.

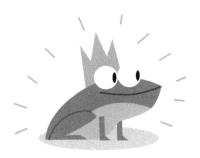

CONTENTS

A Letter to Grown-ups

Parents, caregivers, and guardians, welcome to this book!

My name is April Eldemire. I am a licensed therapist, and I help families communicate better, get along better, and love better. I want families to thrive, not just survive.

ABOUT ME

I earned my bachelor's degree in psychology from Florida State University in 2004, then earned my master's degree in marriage and family therapy from Nova Southeastern University. I am passionate about helping families manage the growing demands of modern parenthood, and my mission is to reach blended families and support them in creating a healthy and loving bond. I am a Bringing Baby Home Educator and wrote a whole series for the internationally recognized Gottman Institute on new-parenthood transitions. I am dedicated to strengthening marriages, families, and relationships.

WHAT I BELIEVE

I believe that home isn't just a place. Home is a feeling that we experience and cultivate while we're around the people we love—including the people we're invited to love when new families are created.

For kids, having somewhere to feel at home is especially important. Home offers the sense of stability, security, and safety that are prerequisites for healthy growth and development. But challenges and conflict can leave kids yearning for what home offers—and perhaps nowhere is this felt more strongly than in families touched by separation, divorce, and remarriage.

That doesn't mean changing family dynamics are all negative, of course. Being a part of a blended family can lead to a number of positive outcomes for both you and your kids.

> *Blended family (noun): a family that includes children of a previous marriage of one spouse or both (Merriam-Webster)*

How can we help our kids hold space for both the negative and positive feelings that invariably arise as a result of their changing family? How can we help them recognize, accept, integrate, and move through what they're feeling—even when what they're feeling is sometimes big, scary, and hard?

WHO THIS BOOK IS FOR—AND WHY IT MATTERS

This book is intended for parents, caregivers, or guardians, and kids (6 to 9 years old) who are adjusting to the novel and changing dynamics of their blended family or who are looking for additional support and tools as they create a sense of home.

Here's why this book matters:

We know that kids of blended families often have emotions that they struggle to make sense of. These can include fear, anger, guilt, sadness, and excitement. (Let's face it: even as adults, *we* sometimes struggle to make sense of these emotions!)

We also know that kids of blended families often have questions that they don't know how to express: *Do my parents still love me? What will my friends think? Will I get along with my stepsiblings?*

Your kids' feelings, thoughts, and actions are normal and to be expected. This book will help your kids learn how to express their feelings in a healthy way and feel safe to ask the questions that might be on their minds.

HOW TO USE THIS BOOK

Inside this book, you'll find dozens of activities that you can do with your kids. These include "on the page" activities, such as writing and art, and "off the page" activities, like breathing or movement exercises. These activities are designed to help kids move through the emotions and challenges they might face as they adjust to their changing family. All of the activity directions are written so your kids can read along with you. And each activity includes a tip for parents and caregivers to adapt the activity as needed or engage in follow-up conversations.

Treat this book as a team-building guide. Do the activities together! You can follow the book in order or pick and choose activities that work best depending on what your child needs at the moment.

Thank you for being here. I am thrilled and honored to share my professional insights and help blended families create a sense of belonging, connection, and clarity in their new homes!

A Letter to Kids

Hello! My name is April. I am a counselor, and I help grown-ups and kids just like you stay strong and feel safe, even when big changes are happening in life.

One big change a lot of kids go through is becoming a part of a blended family. Being in a blended family means that your parents or one of your parents married another grown-up who also has kids. This grown-up is now your stepparent, and their kids are now your stepsiblings. Lucky you—your family just grew!

There are *so many* blended families in the world. Every blended family is special in its own way. Your blended family probably looks different from what your family used to look like, and it's normal to have a lot of tough feelings when you think about the changes your family is going through.

For example, some days you might feel:

- Scared
- Sad
- Mad
- Frustrated
- Nervous
- Confused
- Lonely

It's okay to feel these things. Grown-ups, including your parents, sometimes have these feelings, too. And just like clouds in the sky, these feelings will come and go. Even your biggest, toughest, ickiest feelings don't hang around forever.

By the way, it's normal to have a lot of *good* feelings about your blended family, too—like feeling happy or even excited!

Maybe you're excited to get to know your stepparent and stepsiblings. Maybe you're happy about having a new house to live in or visit. No matter *what* you're feeling about your changing family, it's okay to feel that way.

In this book, you'll find lots of fun activities you can do with your new family. These activities will help you *know* what you're feeling and teach you healthy ways to *show* what you're feeling. The activities even teach you how to use your imagination and your body to turn big, uncomfortable feelings into positive feelings.

There are so many things you can look forward to now that you're part of a blended family. It's time to have fun. Let's get started!

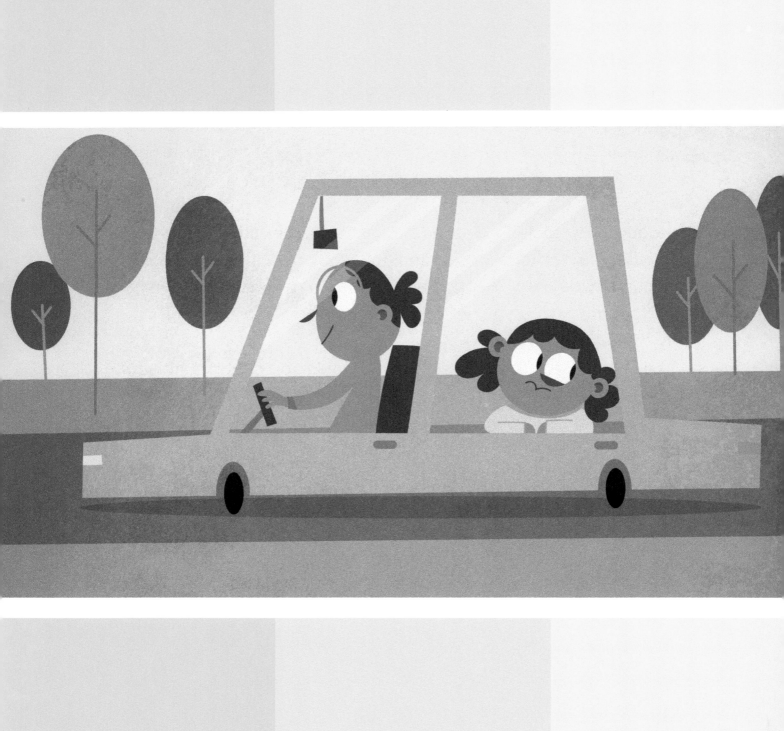

CHAPTER 1

My Family Is Changing

Tanya is six years old. Today, Tanya's mom is driving her over to her dad's new house for the first time. Tanya is going to spend the whole weekend there with her dad and his new wife, Jane, plus Jane's three kids.

"How do you feel about going to spend the weekend at Daddy's house?" Tanya's mom asks.

Tanya is in the back seat of her mom's car. She looks out the window and thinks about it. She then says, "I feel excited to see Daddy and my new room. But I also feel sad because you won't be there. And I feel nervous. What happens if my stepsiblings don't want to play with me?"

Tanya's mother looks at her in the back seat and smiles. "Your stepsiblings will want to play with you, Tanya. You're fun and great at sharing! And it's normal to have all those feelings. Do you want to tell me more?"

INTRODUCTION

When you think about your changing family, what do you think? How do you feel? Do you know it's okay to have those thoughts and feelings—no matter what they are?

Becoming a part of a blended family can lead to a lot of changes in your mind and body. Some days you might feel good, and some days you might feel bad.

Some days you might not even know *what* you're feeling!

The activities in this chapter will help you learn how to pay attention to what you're thinking and feeling as your family changes. When you pay attention to your thoughts and feelings, you will be able to:

◆ Show or tell your feelings in a way that won't hurt yourself or anyone else

◆ Tell someone when you need help

◆ Use your words, body, and imagination to change your feelings from bad to good

Paying attention to what you're feeling and thinking is like being a detective of your own body and mind. It's fun to learn about yourself this way—and the more you understand what's going on inside, the easier it will be to stay strong during the big change that's happening in your family right now.

Let's get started!

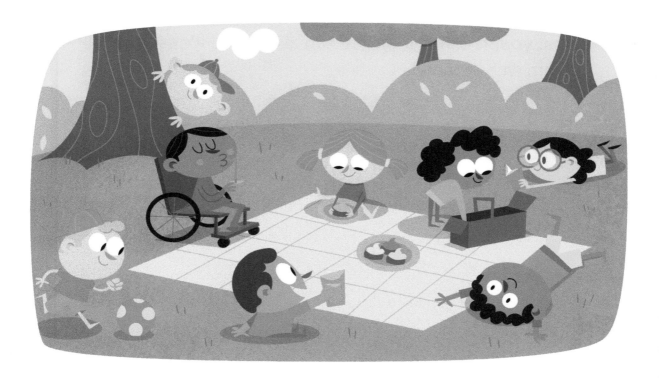

1 DRAW MY FEELINGS

When you have big feelings like sadness or anger, sometimes it can be hard to know what to do with them. One thing you can do is draw your feelings.

Drawing a picture of your feelings means that you get to use your imagination. You can make your feelings look like anything you want!

When you can imagine what your feelings look like, you might be able to notice them more quickly the next time you feel them. Imagining what your feelings look like can also make it easier to talk about them with an adult.

MATERIALS NEEDED

Pens, pencils, crayons, or markers

HOW TO DO THE ACTIVITY ||||||||||||||||||||||||||||||||||||||||||||||||||||||||||||

1. Get your drawing tools.

2. Choose one big feeling you have right now or one you had recently. This might be anger, sadness, or frustration. You can also choose a positive feeling, like happiness or excitement.

3. Use your imagination to draw your feeling in the square. Here are some questions to help you imagine what your feeling might look like:

   a. If your feeling had a color, what would that be? Does it have more than one color?

   b. What shape is your feeling? Is your feeling shaped like an animal, a person, a toy, or something else?

   c. How big is your feeling?

   d. Where does your feeling live?

   e. What does your feeling like to do? Is there anything your feeling *doesn't* like to do?

   f. If your feeling could eat, what do you think its favorite food would be?

Remember, you can make your feeling look like anything you want. You can also draw more than one feeling.

TIPS FOR PARENTS AND CAREGIVERS

You can ask open-ended questions about their drawing instead of making comments or assumptions about the quality of the drawing. So instead of saying, "Wow. That picture looks so scary!" you can try, "I notice you're using a lot of dark colors in your picture. Can you tell me why?" If your child is unable to draw, try modifying this activity by drawing for them while asking them this activity's questions.

LET'S HAVE A PUPPET SHOW!

When you're feeling angry, sad, scared, upset, or some other big emotion, it can be hard to tell someone what you need. Sometimes using your imagination with a puppet or stuffed animal can help you feel safe enough to say what's really on your mind.

With puppets, stuffed animals, or toys, we can also act out challenging moments that happened to us in real life and imagine how we would handle those challenging moments differently if it ever happened again. It's a great way to practice using new words and new actions!

In this activity, we're making puppets and putting on a puppet show. Do this with your whole family so you all can participate.

MATERIALS NEEDED

A clean old sock
Glue
Kid-safe scissors

Arts and craft supplies, like construction paper, googly eyes, markers, pipe cleaners, and string

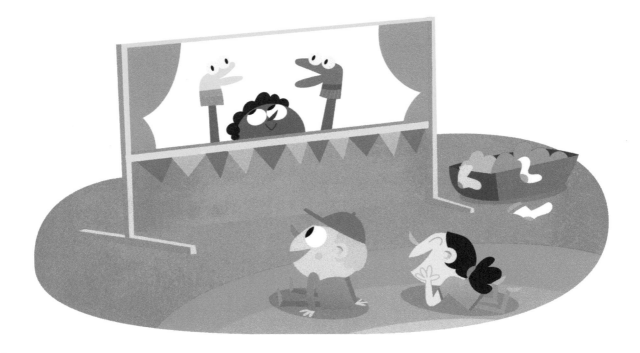

HOW TO DO THE ACTIVITY

1. Gather your art supplies.

2. Put your hand inside your sock (make sure your grown-up knows which sock you are using—you don't want to use one of your best socks!). Move your hand to make it look like the sock is talking. This is your sock puppet!

3. Put your sock back down on the table. Decorate it however you want with the supplies you have. Ask your family members if they would like to make one, too. Once everyone's puppet is done, it's time to put on a puppet show.

4. To start, think about a challenging moment you had with one of your siblings or parents recently, such as an argument or disagreement. Using your puppets, act out how this moment happened in real life as well as you can remember.

5. Next use your imagination and act out this challenging moment in a different way. Think about different words you could say or actions you could do. What happens when you use these new words or behaviors? Does the argument or disagreement end differently? Do you and your siblings feel better?

TIPS FOR PARENTS AND CAREGIVERS

Kids use imagination and play to learn about their world—and learn about themselves. We can encourage our kids to learn how to speak up for themselves while still allowing them to use alternative means of expression as they become more comfortable with this skill.

This might involve letting your kids use a toy or a puppet to "speak" for them. When doing this activity, get on their level, and talk to your kids' puppets directly. Ask open-ended questions, focusing on what your kids were thinking and feeling during this remembered moment. Be sure to encourage your kids to notice what the other kids (and their puppets) are feeling and showing.

3 IT'S TIME FOR A SCAVENGER HUNT OUTSIDE

When you think about your new family, do you ever feel big feelings, like sadness, anger, confusion, or fear? These feelings can be sticky and hard to let go of.

One thing you can do to help calm down is go for a walk or stroll outside. It's even better if you can do this with the whole family. Here's why:

Being outside is a great way to move your body, which is good for your heart, muscles, and bones. Being outside is also a great way to take your mind off stressful thoughts and help you pay more attention to what's going on around you. When you go for a walk or stroll with your grown-ups and stepsiblings, you also get to spend quality time together. This can help you feel more connected and less lonely.

This activity encourages you and your family to take a break and spend time together outside. It doesn't even have to be very far—it can be in your neighborhood or in a nearby park. It includes special scavenger hunts you can do together to take your mind off stressful things and focus on all the cool stuff around you!

MATERIALS NEEDED

Comfortable walking shoes
Sunscreen

Water bottles and snacks

HOW TO DO THE ACTIVITY

1. With your grown-ups and stepsiblings, head outside for a walk or a stroll somewhere if you're able to. Be sure to put on your comfy clothes and wear sunscreen if you need to.

2. While you're outside, use your senses to have a family scavenger hunt. Here are five ideas to get you started (or come up with your own):

    a. Scavenger hunt 1: Find as many animals as you can.

    b. Scavenger hunt 2: Find all the colors of the rainbow—red, orange, yellow, green, blue, and purple.

    c. Scavenger hunt 3: Find as many words (or letters) as you can.

    d. Scavenger hunt 4: Find things that start with the first letter of each person's name in your family.

    e. Scavenger hunt 5: Use your ears to notice as many sounds as you can.

3. Work together to help each other find everything!

TIPS FOR PARENTS AND CAREGIVERS

Going for family walks is a great way for your kids to get to know their new neighborhood (if this applies). As an alternative, consider taking your family for a walk in a familiar place to give them a sense of comfort.

Introducing the scavenger hunt adds a collaborative element to your family work, encouraging you all to work as a team to achieve a goal.

Finally, doing a scavenger hunt also gives your kids an opportunity to practice *mindfulness*—the state of being fully aware and present with what's going on around them. You can be great role models for mindfulness by getting involved in the scavenger hunt and keeping your phone tucked away.

4 THE WHAT-IF GAME

All blended families will have challenging moments from time to time. Maybe you and your siblings don't agree about the rules of a game or you don't want to play the same game. Maybe someone in the family feels left out sometimes or just wants to be alone for a while. Maybe someone, like your teacher or your friend's parent, makes a mistake and thinks your stepparent is your mom or dad. Oops!

Challenges like these are normal when people with different thoughts and experiences come together, spend time with each other, or even live with each other. One good way to prepare for challenges that might show up in your new family is to imagine what they could be and then talk through what everyone could do if those challenges came up in real life.

This activity is a chance for you to use your imagination and work together as a family so you'll be ready for any obstacles that might come your way.

MATERIALS NEEDED

A comfy spot for everyone to get together

Pen or pencil

TIPS FOR PARENTS AND CAREGIVERS

Fostering healthy, dynamic, and interactive communication between your kids and step-kids is a lifelong process. As a blended family, you'll *always* have the opportunity to work on this!

Because you're the grown-ups, consider yourself and your partner as the moderators of this discussion. Make sure each kid gets a chance to speak up. Help your kids realize that there could be more than one correct way to handle each what-if scenario. Each child brings their own experiences and insights to the challenge.

Be sure to add any specific scenarios that have already happened in your lives.

HOW TO DO THE ACTIVITY ||||||||||||||||||||||||||||||||||||||||||||||||||||||||||||||||||

1. Sit down as a family. Read each of the following what-if scenarios.

2. Work together to come up with some ideas for what could be done in each scenario to help everyone feel better.

3. When thinking about what to do in these what-if scenarios, be sure to keep in mind what would be the best ways to help everyone feel safe, heard, and respected.

What should happen if . . .

* Someone doesn't want to share something?

  _____

  _____

* Someone is feeling sad when they come over to the house?

  _____

  _____

* Someone borrows something without asking?

  _____

  _____

* Someone wants to watch a different show or movie than everybody else?

  _____

  _____

* Someone accidentally calls your stepparent your mom or dad?

  _____

  _____

SHAKE, SHAKE, SHAKE

Do you know what ducks do when they get mad?

When ducks get mad, stressed, or scared, or even after they fight with another duck, they usually shake their wings!

Ducks are not shaking their wings to look silly. Shaking their wings helps them get rid of any big energy they have left over from their stressful emotions. They can calm down more quickly and then move on to whatever they're doing next, feeling more relaxed and focused.

Now it's your turn to act like a duck!

This activity teaches you a simple way to help yourself feel better whenever you're feeling upset. You can even use this activity to help yourself calm down after you've had an argument with someone in your family.

MATERIALS NEEDED

Plenty of space to move around   Music (optional)

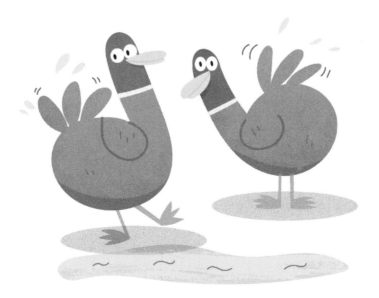

HOW TO DO THE ACTIVITY ||||||||||||||||||||||||||||||||||||||||||||||||||||||

1. Go to a place where you have plenty of room to move around.

2. Take a deep breath. If you'd like, turn on some of your favorite music.

3. Shake, shake, shake your whole body! Shake your head, your arms, your tummy, and your legs, or whatever you are able to. There's no wrong way to shake, as long as you're not bumping into anyone or anything else.

4. While you're shaking, imagine all those bad feelings flying out of your body.

5. You can shake until you feel tired, until your favorite song is over, or until your grown-up says "Stop!" or "Freeze!" You can also try counting to 10 in your head, then stop shaking once you've reached 10.

TIPS FOR PARENTS AND CAREGIVERS

The goal of this activity is to help your kids safely deal with big feelings. With enough practice and reinforcement, your kids may eventually be able to use this strategy without any prompting from you. In the beginning, however, it might be helpful to supervise your child while they're shaking their bodies to ensure they're physically safe and don't inadvertently get themselves worked up again. Be sure to emphasize that shaking is meant to help get big energy and big feelings *out* of their body.

After the exercise, process it with your child. Ask these questions as a guide: What bad feelings did you shake out? How does your body feel after getting rid of those uncomfortable feelings? What made you feel those feelings in the first place?

COOL DOWN OUR BODIES WITH OUR BREATH

Did you know that you breathe more than 20,000 times per day? Breathing is so important because it helps us get oxygen into our bodies—and breathing in certain ways can help us calm down and feel more relaxed.

This activity shows you a great tool you can use the next time you're feeling a big feeling like sadness, anger, fear, or worry. Remember that your feelings are okay to have! Asking a grown-up for help is a really good way to handle your feelings, but it's also great when you can learn how to start making yourself feel better, too.

Wouldn't you like to learn how to make yourself feel better just with your breath?

|||||||||||||||||||||||||||||| **MATERIALS NEEDED** ||||||||||||||||||||||||||||||

None (just a comfortable place to sit or lie down!)

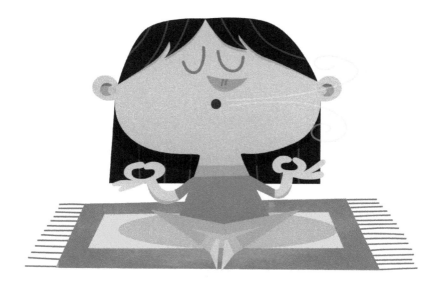

HOW TO DO THE ACTIVITY

1. Find somewhere comfy to sit or lie down. You can close your eyes or keep them open—it's up to you.

2. Take a slow breath in through your nose while thinking, "One, two, three, four."

3. Hold your breath inside your body while thinking, "One, two, three, four."

4. Breathe out through your mouth while thinking, "One, two, three, four."

5. Wait to breathe in again until after you think, "One, two, three, four."

6. Do this 3 times.

TIPS FOR PARENTS AND CAREGIVERS

A highly valuable skill for a child to develop is the ability to recognize when they're having a strong emotion and then knowing how to regulate that emotion on their own. This skill is especially useful when dealing with a major change in the family structure.

Processing this kind of activity helps kids learn about the different events or life changes that make them feel so overwhelmed. Once your child calms down, ask them about the situation so that they can connect the circumstance to the big feeling.

7 POSTURE POWER!

There are three main ways we can communicate with other people: our words (what we say), the tone of our voice (how we make our words sound), and our body language (how we move our face and body). This activity helps you pay attention to the third way you communicate: your body language.

What do your posture and movement say about what you're feeling right now? Let's find out!

Excited	Calm	Happy	Scared	Sad
Confident	Ashamed	Thoughtful	Hurt	Confused
Silly	Proud	Relaxed	Surprised	Disgusted
Worried	Satisfied	Brave	Tired	Thankful
Bored	Angry	Guilty	Jealous	Focused

HOW TO DO THE ACTIVITY ||||||||||||||||||||||||||||||||||||||||||||||||||||||||||||

1. Think about a feeling—let's start with happiness.

2. Imagine what you or someone else looks like when happy.

3. In a mirror or in front of a grown-up, show the feeling of happiness using your body and face. Are you smiling? Waving your arms around? Jumping up and down? Spinning in a circle? You can do whatever feels the most like happiness to you!

4. Now choose another feeling. Let's try sadness. Imagine what you or someone else looks like when they are feeling sad.

5. *Show* the feeling of sadness using your body and face. Are you frowning? Hiding your face behind your hands? Scrunching up into a little ball? Move in whatever way feels the most like sadness to you.

6. Repeat this for as many feelings as you'd like. Use the list of feelings on page 16 and circle them as you do. Do grown-ups or your stepsiblings move in a way that's different from the way you move? It's okay if they do—we all feel our feelings in our own way.

Be sure to move your body in a way that is safe for you and other people around you. For example, it's okay to stomp, but it's not okay to stomp on something and break it!

TIPS FOR PARENTS AND CAREGIVERS

There are so many ways you can modify this posture activity. For example, you can try having your kids take turns showing a particular posture or facial expression and then have the other kids guess what they're feeling. Or ask your kids what sort of feeling they would *like* to have, then encourage them to stand in a way that helps them experience that feeling. This introduces an unexpected but important concept: we can change the way we feel simply by changing the way we hold ourselves or move our bodies.

8 MAKING A WEATHER MAP OF MY FEELINGS

Feelings like happiness, sadness, anger, fear, and loneliness are all normal, especially when you're going through a big change like becoming a part of a blended family. Everyone—including your parents and stepsiblings—has these feelings from time to time.

It's good to remember that even our biggest and toughest feelings are *not* forever. Like clouds in the sky, they will come and go. Just because you might feel bad in one moment doesn't mean you'll feel like that forever. Feelings show up in our bodies, and then they go away when we're done with them. Then another feeling can show up. It's exciting to notice what you'll feel next.

In this activity, you get to pretend that you are a TV weather reporter—but instead of reporting on the weather, you are reporting on your feelings!

MATERIALS NEEDED

Cardstock
Kid-safe scissors
Double-sided Velcro

Drawing utensils, such as colored
pencils, markers, or crayons

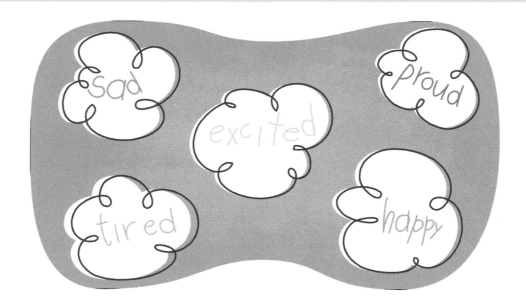

HOW TO DO THE ACTIVITY

1. Cut out clouds from pieces of cardstock. You can make them any shape and size you want.

2. On each cloud, write one feeling—like sad, happy, angry, excited, proud, scared, confused, bored, lonely, or tired.

3. Decorate each cloud however you'd like, using your markers, pens, or pencils. Think about the type of weather that each feeling reminds you of. For example, an angry cloud might look dark and stormy. A happy cloud might be light and fluffy. A sad cloud might look rainy.

4. Cut out 3 to 5 small strips of double-sided Velcro (or ask your grown-up to help). Each strip should have two sides: a rough side (the "hook" side) and a soft side (the "loop" side).

5. Take out another large piece of paper. This is the sky where your clouds will go. You can decorate this paper if you want or just leave it blank.

6. On this large piece of paper, attach the rough sides of your double-sided Velcro.

7. On the back of each cloud, attach the soft side of your double-sided Velcro.

8. Select the cloud that best matches how you're feeling right now, then hang it up in your sky. Feel free to hang more than one cloud if you're noticing more than one feeling inside your body.

TIPS FOR PARENTS AND CAREGIVERS

Have your kids hang this map somewhere they can reach it on their own. This way they can change out the clouds when they want to depending on how they're feeling at the moment. Displaying our maps also encourages kids to be curious about the feelings of the people around them, and it can open up a conversation between siblings and stepsiblings.

FEELING CARDS

When you have big feelings like sadness, anger, and fear, it can be hard to tell or show other people what's going on inside you. But being able to tell others what's going on inside can help you feel better, and sharing the feelings you're noticing can make them seem less big and scary.

This activity will show you how to describe what you're feeling to other people. You'll use a deck of cards that you get to make yourself!

MATERIALS NEEDED

Index cards

Drawing utensils, such as colored pencils, markers, or crayons

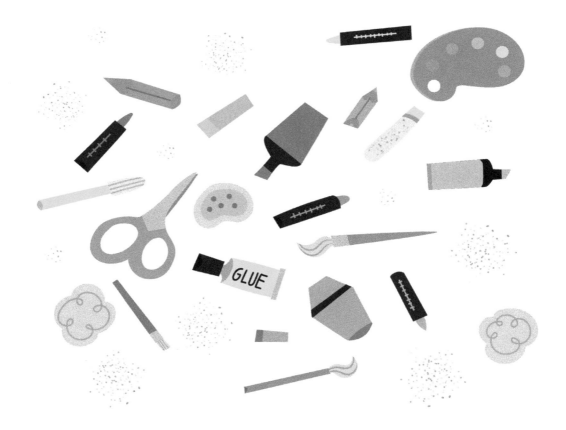

HOW TO DO THE ACTIVITY |||||||||||||||||||||||||||||||||||||||||||||||||||||||||||||

1. Gather all your drawing materials.

2. On one side of an index card, write down the word "sad." If you need to, ask your grown-up for help with this part.

3. On the other side of the card, draw whatever shapes, images, or pictures come to mind when you think about the feeling sad. Use your imagination!

4. Make another card for every feeling you can think of, like angry, happy, scared, frustrated, lonely, excited, tired, or nervous.

5. You now have a whole deck of feeling cards! The next time you're feeling something, you can find the card that matches what you're feeling and show it to your grown-up.

TIPS FOR PARENTS AND CAREGIVERS

It's not always easy for kids to describe what they're feeling—especially when they're very upset or actively crying. Let your kids know that these cards can be a helpful tool for communicating what they're feeling, particularly when they're having a hard time putting things into words.

Encourage your kids to keep these cards in a special place that's easy to get to. Then the next time they seem to be struggling with an emotion, you can prompt them with a phrase such as, "You look like you're having a big feeling. Can you go get your feeling cards and show me which one matches what's going on inside your body right now?"

10 MOVE LIKE AN ANIMAL

Moving makes your body feel good. It can also be a great way to express how you're feeling. Sometimes it's even more fun to move like animals!

The feelings we have might remind us of certain animals. For example, what animal comes to mind when you think of the feeling anger? Maybe you think of a lion roaring, or a gorilla pounding its chest, or an elephant stomping on the ground. Or maybe you think of a different animal altogether.

What about when you think of the feeling happiness? Do you think of a dog wagging its tail, a bird flying, or a kitten playing with a ball of string?

What animal comes to mind when you think of the feeling scared? Do you think of a mouse hiding in its nest? Do you think of a bunny hopping away?

This activity helps you think about what you're feeling inside and then expressing it in a fun way—by moving like an animal!

MATERIALS NEEDED

Space to move around   Music (optional)

HOW TO DO THE ACTIVITY

1. Think of a big feeling you're having now or had recently.

2. Next think of an animal that reminds you of how you feel or felt.

3. Now, move like that animal!

TIPS FOR PARENTS AND CAREGIVERS

Don't be surprised if your kids think of different animals while working on the same emotion. Remind your kids that every person feels their emotions a little differently and there's no "right" or "wrong" answer.

To help prompt your kids, you can start by naming the animal—try a wide range, like dog, cat, frog, snake, elephant, gorilla, lion, fish, and bird. Next ask your child to move like that animal and then to reflect on what feeling their movements reminds them of. This is another great activity that helps kids understand that the way they *feel* can change the way they *move*—and the way they *move* can also change the way they *feel*.

Be sure to join in the fun and do this right along with the family!

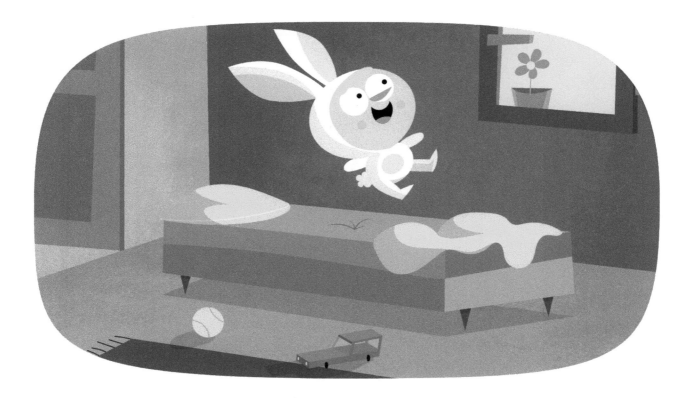

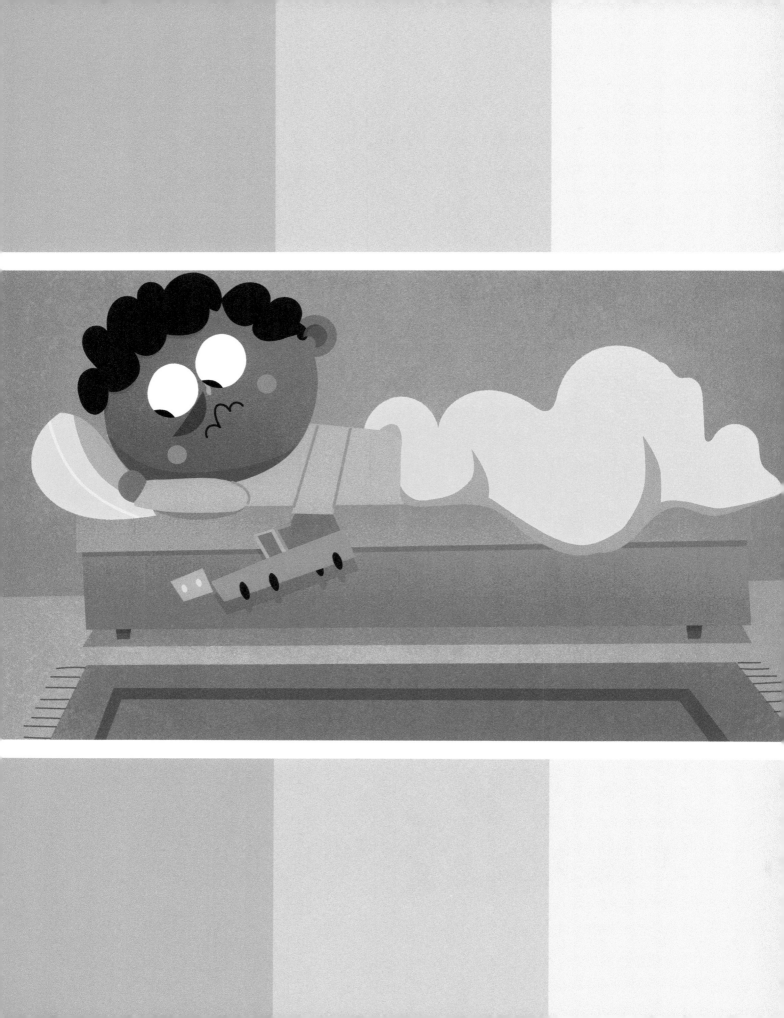

CHAPTER 2

Feeling My Feelings Is Hard

Jason walks into his stepbrother Sam's room and sees Sam sitting on the floor. Sam has an angry look on his face, and he is smashing his toy trucks together.

"Are you okay, Sam?" Jason asks.

Sam looks up from the floor with a frown. "I'm mad!" he yells.

"Why are you mad?" Jason asks.

Sam drops his toys and jumps up onto his bed. He rolls on his side, facing away from Jason. "I don't know why. I just *am*," he growls. "Now leave me alone!"

Jason walks away and finds his mom. He tells her what happened and asks her why Sam is so upset.

"It looks like you're feeling sad about how Sam spoke to you," his mom says. "I can understand why you would feel that way. Sam has been having some big feelings, too, ever since moving into our house with your stepdad. I want you to know that it's not okay Sam yelled at you, but it is okay for him to feel mad sometimes. Just like it's okay for you to feel sad. We need to help each other learn how to show our feelings in ways that won't hurt ourselves or other people."

INTRODUCTION

When your family goes through big changes, it's normal to feel a *lot* of different emotions or feelings, such as:

◆ Happy

◆ Sad

◆ Angry

◆ Confused

◆ Scared

◆ Lonely

Some of these emotions might feel good—and some of these emotions might not feel good. But no matter what emotions you're feeling at any moment, it's important to remember that it's okay for you to feel them. Really!

Even the emotions that don't feel very good, like anger or sadness, are allowed to be there. In fact, *all* of your emotions are important and normal, especially when your family is changing or growing.

Emotions are like clouds floating through the sky—they will come, and then they will go. Being able to feel these different emotions is one of the best parts of being *you*. Plus, when you can talk about what you're feeling inside, you'll be able to tell other people what you need—like a hug, some quiet time alone, some help, or something else.

Remember: Even grown-ups and superheroes feel "bad" sometimes. And what will make *you* feel like a superhero is being able to show and talk about your feelings in a way that doesn't hurt other people or yourself.

The activities in this chapter are fun ways to help you:

- Know the emotions or feelings you have inside

- Understand that it's okay for your feelings to exist—even if they are tricky and big!

- Talk about your feelings with other people, including grown-ups

- Notice your negative thoughts and turn them around

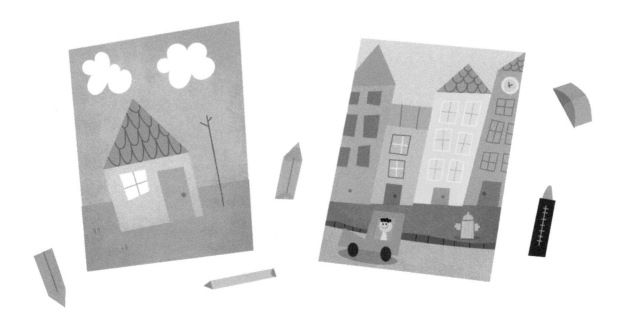

HOME SWEET HOMES!

Can you call more than one place home?

Maybe you lived in one house with your parents for a long time. Now you're living in two separate homes that seem different and strange and filled with new people. Maybe all these changes are bringing up a lot of different emotions.

It's okay to have all these feelings about your new homes. In this activity, you get to sit down, draw your homes, and put your family inside the drawings. You'll see that you really do belong in both places!

MATERIALS NEEDED

Drawing utensils, such as colored pencils, markers, or crayons

1. Use your imagination to draw a picture in the drawing space on page 28 of the two homes you live in now.

2. While drawing your two homes, think about what they look like. Think about the types of furniture, paint, and rooms that are inside each home. Imagine the smells, sounds, colors, and materials. Who lives in each of these homes? Be sure to add the people, including yourself.

3. As you draw each of your homes, add in things that bring you comfort. Maybe you want to include a stack of books or your favorite arts and crafts supplies. Create an image of your new homes with all the things inside that you love.

4. When you're done drawing your homes, share them with your family. Point to the parts of your homes where you find yourself feeling nervous, worried, or unsure. Then point to the parts of your homes where you feel the most "at home," comfortable, excited, or relaxed. Does anyone else feel the same way?

TIPS FOR PARENTS AND CAREGIVERS

Establishing a sense of "home base" is so important for your kids to feel relaxed, comfortable, and secure in their new home (or homes). Being able to conceptualize what their homes look like helps your children start to feel like they "fit in" to a new space.

If your child struggles to identify a specific area of your home where they feel the most relaxed or comfortable, use this activity as an opportunity to cocreate a space that feels inviting and calming to them. Maybe you can redecorate a room together, or hang out in that area more often, or put some of their favorite comfort items in that area.

DIVE INTO THE DEEP END OF THE POOL

The shallow end of the swimming pool is for wading and playing games like Marco Polo. The deep end of the pool is where you can jump in, swim, or do a cannonball (if you're a good swimmer).

Picturing a pool can be a helpful way to think about and work through our emotions. Talking about what we're feeling is like wading in the shallow end of the pool. Figuring out *why* we're feeling what we're feeling is like diving deeper.

In this activity, we'll use our imagination to "swim with our emotions" and start to figure out why different emotions come up.

MATERIALS NEEDED

None (just a comfy spot to sit and think!)

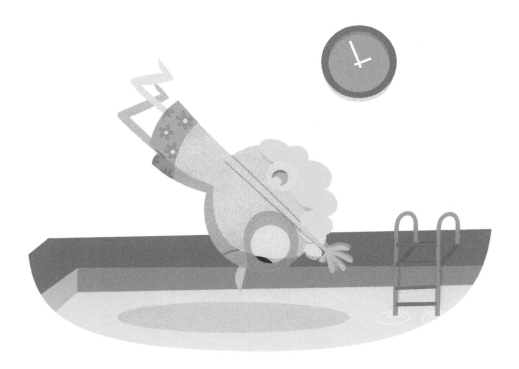

HOW TO DO THE ACTIVITY

1. Close your eyes and imagine that you're stepping into a pool. Feel your toes in the water.

2. Use your imagination to see feelings floating around in the shallow end of the pool, just like pool toys or rubber ducks. Look around the pool until you see a feeling that you've been having lately about your changing family—such as sad, mad, angry, lonely, or scared. See yourself wading over to the feeling and holding on to it.

3. In your imagination, take your feeling and swim to the deep end. Take a deep breath and dive underwater with your feeling.

4. As you dive underwater in your imagination, ask yourself, "Why do I have this feeling? What could it be?" Listen to the answer that comes up. Maybe you're feeling guilty because you miss one parent and not the other. Perhaps you're feeling anxious or scared because one of your new homes is busy and full of new people. Maybe you're feeling angry because your parent said they were too busy to play with you. It's okay if there's more than one answer. It's also okay if you listen but still don't hear any answer at all.

5. Now it's time to swim back to the surface. In your imagination, come up for air. Take a big, deep breath, look at your feeling, and say, "It's okay to feel this." Then, when you're ready, you can let go of your feeling and watch it float away.

TIPS FOR PARENTS AND CAREGIVERS

Diving deep and tapping into the root of your emotions can be scary—just like diving into the deep end of the pool can be scary. For this visualization exercise, help your kids imagine the scene in a way that makes them feel safe. For instance, if they don't know how to swim, you can help them picture themselves wearing floaties or a life vest.

It might be helpful to read this activity aloud to your child so they can simply close their eyes and focus on their imagination. Be there to check in with them and talk about what they're experiencing.

13 LICK A LOLLIPOP!

Have you ever licked a Tootsie Pop?

The outside of the lollipop is sweet and sticky. But as you keep licking, eventually you get to the center of the lollipop, which is chocolaty and gooey. Getting to the center of the lollipop is so fun!

Sitting down and thinking about our feelings can be a lot like licking a Tootsie Pop. That's because sometimes what we're feeling on the *outside* is different from what we're really feeling deep on the *inside*.

For example, maybe sometimes you look and feel angry. You stomp your feet or scrunch up your eyebrows. But if you get quiet and think about where your anger came from, you might realize that beneath your anger is another feeling, like sadness.

This activity uses a tasty treat to help us peel back the layers of our emotions and identify what we're really feeling inside.

MATERIALS NEEDED

A Tootsie Pop lollipop (or another tasty treat)

HOW TO DO THE ACTIVITY

1. Sit down with your favorite flavor Tootsie Pop—yum!

2. As you lick your lollipop, think about a recent situation at home that made you have a big feeling. Maybe it was having to share a room with your stepsibling. Maybe you couldn't find the toy you wanted because you left it at your other house. What was the big feeling you had? Can you name it? Were you frustrated, angry, or annoyed?

3. Once you've named your feeling, keep licking. Look at your lollipop and watch it change. Keep thinking about that situation. Just like your lollipop changes inside, so can your feelings. What else did you feel? Were you sad? Worried? Confused?

4. As you enjoy your special treat, talk with a grown-up about all the feelings you notice.

TIPS FOR PARENTS AND CAREGIVERS

Both adults and kids sometimes struggle to remember that even uncomfortable emotions are meant to be brought to light and understood—and that we often feel more than one uncomfortable feeling at once.

The thing is, once we figure out all the different emotions we're experiencing, we can advocate for our needs better and express ourselves in a more appropriate and functional way. This activity is meant to help your kid see that all the emotions they feel are normal and the first emotion they identify might not actually be what's really at "the center of the Tootsie Pop." Kick back and enjoy this treat with them—and enjoy discovering your diverse realm of emotions, too!

If your child has an allergy or dietary restriction, considering modifying this activity and replacing the lollipop with another food that has many layers.

14 INTERVIEW YOURSELF!

When your family is going through a big change, it can be hard to remember that you deserve to feel good about yourself—no matter what emotions you're feeling. But when you're feeling big feelings like anger or sadness, it can be hard to feel close to the person you are inside.

In this activity, you get to sit down and ask yourself some questions. Just like people interview celebrities and athletes so we can get to know them better, we can "interview" ourselves and get to know ourselves better, too.

MATERIALS NEEDED

Pen or pencil

TIPS FOR PARENTS AND CAREGIVERS

You can help guide your children through this journaling activity whether they're able to write or not. For example, depending on your child's ability, it might be more appropriate for them to type out their answers on a computer, use a talk-to-text app, or even record their voice. Or perhaps you'd rather sit down together and just talk through these questions in a more conversational style.

Self-reflection activities like this help children understand that they have their own unique ways of responding to their emotions—and that other people might feel the same way but act very differently.

HOW TO DO THE ACTIVITY

1. Write down your answers to each of the following questions:

   ◆ What do I do when I'm feeling scared?

   _____

   _____

   ◆ Who do I talk to when I'm sad?

   _____

   _____

   ◆ How do I express my anger?

   _____

   _____

   ◆ Do I hide my emotions inside or let them out?

   _____

   _____

   ◆ What helps me calm down when I'm feeling overwhelmed?

   _____

   _____

   ◆ When I'm hurting, what do I say to myself?

   _____

   _____

   ◆ When do I feel the most loved and accepted?

   _____

   _____

   ◆ What things do I do that I am the proudest of?

   _____

   _____

   ◆ How do I wish others would see me?

   _____

   _____

   ◆ When do I doubt myself?

   _____

   _____

2. Discuss your answers with your parents and/or stepsiblings.

TIMBER! BUILDING A TOWER OF EMOTIONS

Have you ever gotten very angry very quickly at someone in your family "out of nowhere"?

The truth is, our emotions don't come from nowhere. They always tell the truth about what's going on inside our bodies. But sometimes our big feelings can build up slowly. Small things that happen or small things that other people do might cause a feeling to start growing inside you. When the feeling is still small, you might not notice it right away. Maybe you just feel a little "off" or you have a bellyache.

If you don't notice your feeling right away, it can get bigger and bigger, especially if other things continue to happen that annoy or frustrate you. Your feeling gets bigger . . . and bigger . . . until it is *so* big that you want to yell, cry, scream, or run!

Of course, it's not a bad thing to have big feelings—but it's not okay to express your big feelings in a way that is destructive or harmful. The good news is, the sooner you can recognize your feelings, *even when they are still small*, the sooner you can express how you feel and tell other people what you need.

In this activity, you get some free play with blocks to see what happens when you allow things to slowly build up over time.

MATERIALS NEEDED

Blocks that you are allowed to
  write on

Marker
Sticky notes

TIPS FOR PARENTS AND CAREGIVERS

This activity is a good visual for helping kids see the impact of letting emotions "pile up" inside them. Be sure to supervise your kids while doing this activity, since falling blocks may be hazardous. These blocks can also be reused for activity 46.

1. Lay out all your blocks, or whatever you're using for building material.

2. Write the name of a different emotion or feeling on each block (or write them on sticky notes and stick them to the blocks). Include as many emotions as you can. Include emotions that feel good and ones that feel bad. Examples are: sad, mad, angry, confused, scared, anxious, happy, excited, lonely, irritated, and upset. You can put the same emotion on more than one block. It's up to you!

3. Once you have labeled all your blocks, start stacking them up one by one.

4. Notice what happens when your block stack has only a few blocks. Is it sturdy? If you gently tap your finger against the stack, does it tip over?

5. Keep piling up your feeling blocks one by one. As the stack gets taller, what happens to it? Does it look more steady or less steady? What happens when you gently tap your finger against the stack? Does it tip?

6. At some point, your stack of feeling blocks might build up so high that it starts to sway and wobble. It might even fall over with a loud crash. This is just like what can happen when we let our feelings pile up inside us.

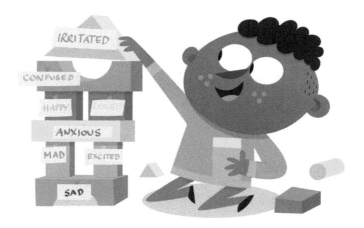

When we have big feelings that feel uncomfortable, our bodies often respond by trying to be fast: we breathe fast, we move fast, we think fast, and we fidget and fuss. It might feel strange, but slowing down our bodies and minds can often help feelings get smaller on their own and eventually go away. SLOW is a good way to remember some of the biggest feelings we have when our families change: Sad, Lonely, Overwhelmed, and Worried. The next time you have any of these big feelings, use this tracing activity to help yourself calm down and slow down.

||||||||||||||||||||||||||||||| **MATERIALS NEEDED** |||||||||||||||||||||||||||||||

| Drawing utensils, such as colored pencils, markers, or crayons | A favorite toy that you can hold in your hand |

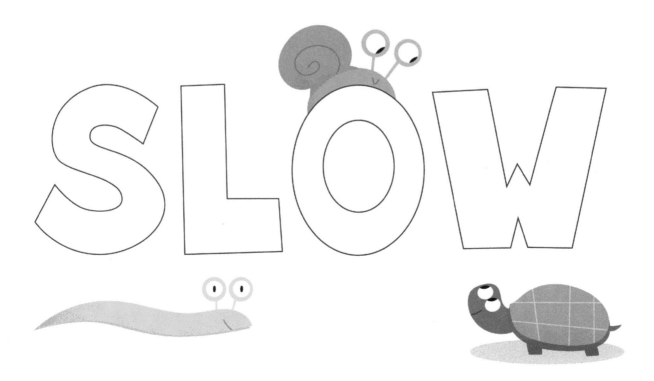

HOW TO DO THE ACTIVITY

1. Feel free to add colors, decorations, and pictures to the letters in the word *SLOW* on page 38.

2. Get a favorite toy. You can use anything you want as long as it's small enough to fit in your hand. Examples are toy cars, toy trains, or even a small stuffed animal.

3. Use your toy to slowly trace each letter in the word *SLOW*, starting with the letter S. Make it a game—how slowly can your toy move? Can you move slower than a turtle, a sloth, or a slug? Can you move like you are in slow motion?

4. As you trace the word *SLOW* with your toy, take slow, deep breaths.

5. When you're done tracing the word *SLOW*, put your toy down. Notice how your body and mind feel. Do they feel any different?

TIPS FOR PARENTS AND CAREGIVERS

The goal of this activity is grounding: to help your child slow down, direct their attention, and use their breath and deliberate, present-minded action to regulate their nervous system and soothe themselves.

Your kids can do this activity anywhere, anytime—even if they don't have a piece of paper handy. Teach them to use their finger to trace out the word *SLOW* on the palm of their hand or on a table.

What does *extreme* mean? Extreme means something that is as far away from ordinary as it can get.

Deserts are some of the hottest and driest places on earth. They get less than a foot of rainfall each year and are an example of an extreme part of the world. Rain forests are also extreme but in the opposite way. Rain forests are very wet and can get more than six feet of rainfall per year!

Sometimes being in a blended family can feel extreme, too. On some days, everyone seems to get along and you might have a lot of great feelings. Other days, people might feel tense or angry.

When things at home feel extreme, you can find comfort in knowing that the extreme situations in your home won't last forever—and even in extreme situations, beautiful things can be found.

MATERIALS NEEDED

Books about deserts and rain forests	Internet resources Pen or pencil

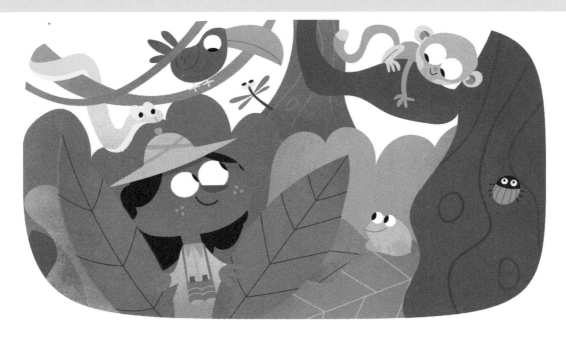

HOW TO DO THE ACTIVITY ||||||||||||||||||||||||||||||||||||||||||||||||||||||||||||||

With a grown-up's permission, use the internet, library books, and other resources to start researching facts about deserts and rain forests. Even though these two parts of the earth are very extreme and different from each other, they are both home to some pretty amazing things! List out 10 animals and 5 plants that live in desert and rainforest environments.

TIPS FOR PARENTS AND CAREGIVERS

This educationally oriented activity is a metaphor for the diverse and complex ecosystem that is your blended family. Even in extreme environments—as we often find in families who are adjusting to their new dynamics—good things can come, and growth is constantly occurring. Helping your kid start to see their new family "like a rain forest" or even "like a desert" can help them learn to see all the beautiful things they can look forward to.

Desert Animals	Rain Forest Animals
1.	1.
2.	2.
3.	3.
4.	4.
5.	5.
6.	6.
7.	7.
8.	8.
9.	9.
10.	10.
Desert Plants	**Rain Forest Plants**
1.	1.
2.	2.
3.	3.
4.	4.
5.	5.

18

LET'S PRETEND: PARTS OF A TREE

Look at a tree outside. Can you see all of it?

No—not even if you're standing right in front of it! That's because deep below the ground are the tree's roots, which are the strongest part of the tree. Even though we don't see them, the roots are very important for helping the tree grow and stand strong.

The leaves on a tree are important, too. Leaves turn sunshine into food for the tree so it can keep growing. But unlike roots, leaves can shake in the wind and even fall off.

Just like a tree, you have lots of different parts. Your feelings are a lot like leaves because they can move and go away. And just like leaves on a tree come and go with every season, you'll have new feelings come and go depending on the season of your life.

Your body is a lot like the roots of a tree. Even when your feelings change, your body is still there, growing strong.

MATERIALS NEEDED

Space to move your body   Music

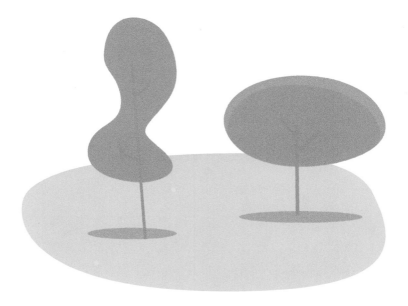

HOW TO DO THE ACTIVITY |||||||||||||||||||||||||||||||||||||||||||||||||||||||||||||||||

1. Put on some comfy clothes and find a space to move around. Ask a grown-up to play your favorite music while you do this activity.

2. As the music plays, move your body in a way that matches a certain emotion. Start with the emotion *happy*. How do you show someone you're happy? What ways might you move your body when you're feeling happy? Go ahead and show us!

3. When your grown-up pauses the music, stop. Picture yourself being strong and tall, like a tree with deep roots.

4. When your grown-up starts the music again, start moving in a way that matches the emotion *angry*. How do you show someone you're angry? What ways might you move your body when you're feeling angry? Be sure to show us in a way that does not hurt yourself, other things, or other people.

5. When your grown-up pauses the music, stop. Picture yourself being strong and tall again, like a tree.

6. Repeat this activity, using as many different emotions as you want. Notice that no matter what kind of feeling you show, you can always come back to stillness in your body—just like the strong roots of a tree are always there, even as leaves grow and fall off the branches.

TIPS FOR PARENTS AND CAREGIVERS

This physical exercise is intended to help kids understand that no matter what they're feeling, it doesn't change who they are inside. This activity also taps into the idea that our posture or positioning can actually influence how we feel inside. Standing or sitting in a tall, confident pose if you are able to can actually help us *feel* more confident.

Encourage your kids to be creative about how they can stand "like a tree"—maybe they can stand with their hands over their head or on their hips, or with their feet wide, or however else their unique body moves.

19

MAKE YOUR OWN SUPERHERO SHIELD!

Sometimes you might notice yourself thinking about the past or worrying about the future. Everybody does this from time to time.

But your imagination is more powerful than you think. When you repeatedly think about things that you're scared of or worried about, they can actually start to feel bigger and more difficult to handle.

The good news is, we can learn how to use our powerful brains to make things feel less scary, too! In fact, if you were a superhero, your imagination would be one of your best superpowers.

In this activity, you'll get to use the real-life superpower of your imagination to help you deal with your negative thoughts.

MATERIALS NEEDED

A large piece of cardboard
  or poster board
Kid-safe scissors
Arts and crafts supplies, such
  as paint, stickers, markers, or
  whatever else you'd like to use

Staples, glue, or strong tape
Two straps of sturdy fabric, about
  12 inches long and 4 inches wide

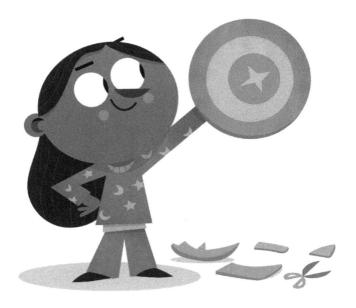

HOW TO DO THE ACTIVITY

1. Cut your piece of cardboard or poster board into the shape of a shield—any shape you'd like. If you need to, ask your grown-up for help.

2. Using your arts and crafts supplies, decorate your shield. Think of words, colors, shapes, objects, or images that make you really feel like a superhero, and put them on your shield. Think about some of your favorite superheroes for ideas.

3. Once the front of your shield is done and dry, carefully turn it over. Using staples, glue, or sturdy tape, attach the strips of fabric to the back. Attach the ends of each strip of fabric so you have two loops lined up with each other. The first loop should be large enough to slip your arm through. The second loop should be big enough for you to hold in your hand. Now you can carry your shield!

Many superheroes use shields to protect them as they face down big challenges, and now you have your very own! The next time you start to notice negative feelings in your mind, pick up your shield. See if you can use your imagination to pretend that you're a tall, strong superhero facing the big challenge of a scary or worrisome thought. Think about how a superhero would look. Can you show us that? Go ahead and act it out! Do you feel any different after you put the shield down?

Know that it's safe to talk about your negative thoughts (even without your shield) and that by doing so, you can help those thoughts quiet down and be less tricky.

TIPS FOR PARENTS AND CAREGIVERS

This activity encourages your kids to "be their own superhero," and it gives them a practical tool—the shield—to really get into the habit of facing down their own challenging thoughts. Your support and guidance remain important as your kids learn to address their negative thinking, but this type of activity can help them learn how to do more of it on their own.

20 A SPECIAL SPOT TO SIT WITH MY FEELINGS

Kids and grown-ups both struggle with tough and challenging emotions, which can have a big impact on their friendships and relationships. We might say things like, "I can't do that," "I don't know how to stop being angry," or "I won't ever like my new life."

It's normal to feel like you don't have control over your feelings, especially when they're difficult ones, such as feeling sad, mad, or scared. Are you sad that you don't like your new stepdad? Are you mad that it isn't just you and your mom anymore? Are you scared about the future and how it will turn out? The more we struggle with these uncomfortable feelings, the worse they become, and the harder they are to let go.

This activity helps you create a place in your home where you can sit, snuggle up, and relax when you have big feelings. When your body feels safe, you'll feel safe to let your feelings move through you.

MATERIALS NEEDED

Blankets, pillows, stuffed animals, and other comfort items

HOW TO DO THE ACTIVITY

1. Create a special spot in your room where you can sit and relax the next time you have a big feeling. This could be in a corner, on your bed, or even in the closet. If you share a room with your stepsiblings or siblings, make sure they're okay with the space you choose. Your parents can help!

2. Make this space as comfy as possible. Add pillows, blankets, stuffed animals, a squeezy stress ball, a box of tissues, or even a bottle of water. If you can, hang some nice pictures or pretty lights nearby—anything you need to make it feel like a safe, relaxing space.

3. The next time you're at home and you have a tricky big feeling, head on over to your special spot. You can even say to your family, "I'm going to go sit in my special spot." Here, you can just sit with your feelings and let them be. It's okay if you cry, take deep breaths, or just think about what's going on in your body. When you're ready, go to your grown-up and talk about what made you want to go sit with your feelings in your special space.

TIPS FOR PARENTS AND CAREGIVERS

All of us, and especially kids, deserve the chance to just express and work through our emotions. To do this successfully and efficiently, it helps to have a space where we can feel safe to process what's going on inside. Helping your kids establish their own special spot can also help them feel more at home in their new environment.

This is entirely different from the more traditional "time-out." The goal with this activity is to help your kids *voluntarily* seek out a quiet space when they're struggling. You can support them by asking questions like, "You're crying and having a hard time telling me what's going on. Did you want to go sit in your special spot for a while until you feel better?" Do not force them to go to their special spot if they don't want to; this space should feel like a refuge that offers a sense of peace and comfort.

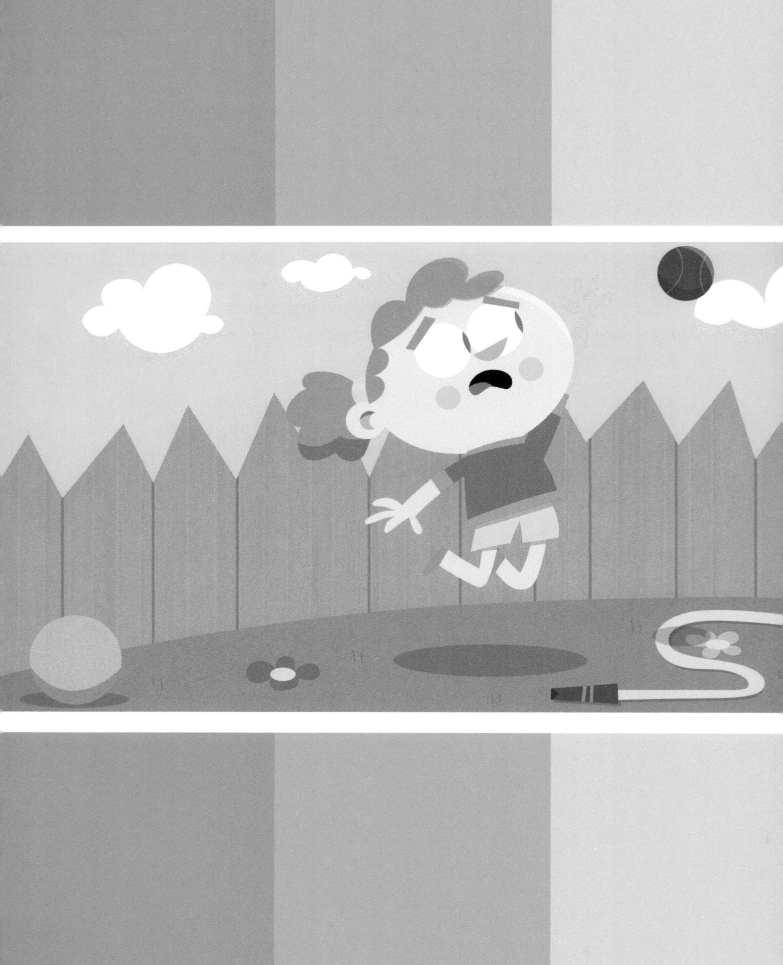

CHAPTER 3

Loving Myself Will Help Me Love My Family

Harriet is at her mom and stepdad's house. She walks outside and sees her stepsiblings, Jess and Tina, playing catch with their mitts and a baseball.

"Hey, Harriet," they say, waving her over. "Come play with us!"

Harriet runs over, excited to play—until she realizes she doesn't have a baseball mitt.

"Don't worry," Jess says, "We'll toss the ball a little slower to you so you can catch it."

But even with her stepsiblings throwing the ball more slowly, Harriet *still* drops the ball—three times in a row!

Harriet holds back tears. "I'm so bad at this," she says, scuffing her foot against the ground.

Jess and Tina look at each other. They walk over and put their arms around Harriet. "Don't be so hard on yourself, Harriet. You're so fun to play with! Let's play something else. What do you want to do?"

INTRODUCTION

Do you ever feel sad, scared, embarrassed, frustrated, or angry? It's normal to have big feelings like these—everybody does. The tricky thing about big feelings is that they can make us forget about all the great things we like about ourselves.

Here's a little secret: loving yourself and remembering your good qualities, even when you feel bad, is like a superpower!

We're extra lucky when we're surrounded by people we love—or even new family members we are learning to love. They remind us of all the good things about ourselves when we're feeling down, just like what Tina and Jess did for Harriet.

If it's hard to feel good about yourself when you're having big feelings, you're not alone. Grown-ups struggle with this, too. Just remember that the person you are on the inside doesn't stop being lovable when your emotions are tough.

The activities in this chapter are fun ways to help you:

◆ Find ways to show yourself love and care

◆ Enjoy more of the activities that *you* really like!

◆ Be brave, even when you're not feeling very loved or lovable

◆ Learn how being kind to yourself helps you be kind to your families

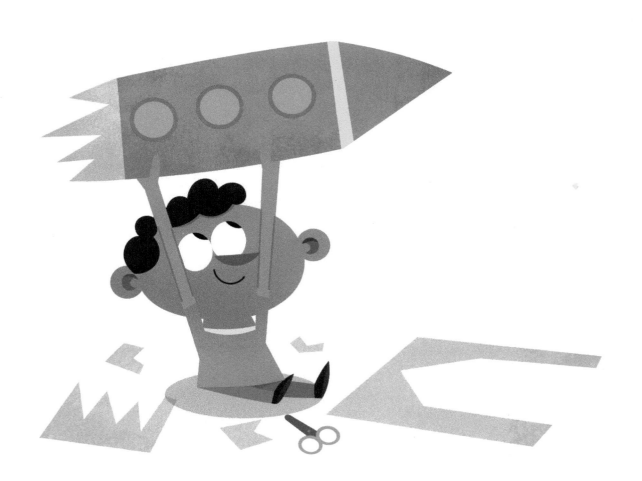

21 | A THANK-YOU NOTE TO MYSELF!

It's polite to say "thank you" when someone is helpful or does something nice. And when you *really* want to show someone appreciation, it's even nicer to write them a thank-you note.

Here's a question: Have you ever written a thank-you note to *yourself*?

It might sound silly, but writing a thank-you note to yourself can be a great way to remember all the good things you do to take care of yourself every day. After all, it's easy to show others that we appreciate them and all the wonderful things they do. I say it's time you start showing yourself some appreciation, too!

MATERIALS NEEDED

Pen or pencil
Paper

(If you prefer, you can also do this on a computer or whatever device you use.)

TIPS FOR PARENTS AND CAREGIVERS

While parents and caregivers are encouraged to join in all the activities in this workbook, this activity in particular is one that I strongly recommend. As grown-ups, we all know how hard it can be to keep from getting down on ourselves when we're feeling strong emotions. A thank-you note to yourself is a powerful way to reflect on your own strengths and quiet that inner critic.

Be prepared to offer up plenty of suggestions to your kids if they're struggling to find things about themselves to be thankful for. They deserve to celebrate themselves every once in a while!

HOW TO DO THE ACTIVITY ||||||||||||||||||||||||||||||||||||||||||||||||||||||||||||||||||||

1. Sit down in a comfy spot with your writing utensils.

2. Start your thank-you note to yourself with the words, "Dear [your name]," just like you would if you were writing it to someone else.

3. Spend at least 10 minutes writing down all the things about yourself that you're thankful for. Maybe you're thankful to yourself for eating food that makes you healthy, or for being kind to your siblings and stepsiblings, or for working so hard in school. Perhaps you're thankful for trying again after you made a mistake. Maybe you're thankful for how you acted in a specific moment from your past. What about yourself makes you the most glad?

Be as creative as you'd like. There is *so* much about yourself that you can feel thankful for!

_____

_____

_____

_____

_____

_____

_____

_____

_____

_____

22 THE TALKING MIRROR

When you look in the mirror, what do you see?

Even if you see some things you don't like, I'll bet you can find way more things that you *do* like. Maybe you love your hair, or the shape of your nose, or the color of your eyes, or your freckles, or the strength of your shoulders. Maybe you love your height, or your style of clothing, or the way you dance to your favorite tunes!

Looking in the mirror isn't just good for fixing your hairdo or finding that spinach to pick out from between your teeth. Scientists know that when you spend time gazing at yourself in the mirror, you can actually:

◆ Learn how to stay in the moment and keep your mind from worrying about the future quite so much

◆ Decrease stress

◆ Increase the love you feel for yourself

Let's take a look at the cool person looking back at you in the mirror!

MATERIALS NEEDED	
A mirror—any size will do, but it's best to find one big enough to see your whole face	A clock, a phone, or anything with a timer

HOW TO DO THE ACTIVITY

1. Stand or sit comfortably in front of your mirror.

2. Set a timer for 2 minutes.

3. Look at your reflection until the timer goes off. (This might seem like a *really* long time—most of us don't stand in front of a mirror for that long!) While you're looking at yourself, feel free to pay close attention to details in your reflection, like the specks of color in your eyes or the way your mouth can move in different ways. It's so interesting to really *look* at who you are.

4. If you feel comfortable, try talking to your reflection. Maybe pretend that your reflection is a friend sitting in front of you who is about to do something challenging. What would you say to them? "You can do this!" "You are strong!" "You are creative!" Be as kind, supportive, and loving as you can.

TIPS FOR PARENTS AND CAREGIVERS

I find this exercise to be especially useful because so many of us use mirrors to fixate on all our "flaws." Learning how to love what they see in the mirror can help your child stay self-loving, even when things are challenging.

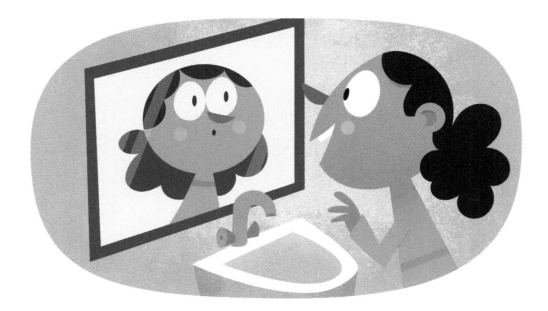

23 | WORD SWAP

The words you say aloud and in your head can make a big difference in your life—and other people's lives, too. Words can help you feel big, brave, strong, and caring, or they can make you feel small, scared, angry, and lonely.

Words are important! But sometimes we don't always think about the words we say, especially when we're feeling bad.

In this activity, you get to practice paying attention to the things you say, and you'll choose different words to help you stay more loving and strong.

MATERIALS NEEDED

Pen or pencil

TIPS FOR PARENTS AND CAREGIVERS

This activity is a great brainteaser. In addition to exploring the phrases presented here, try thinking about a phrase that your child, or anyone in your family, might say frequently, and try to come up with a positive word swap.

When we teach our kids early in life that their words really do shape their experiences, we help them grow into self-compassionate, responsible, and assertive people who can communicate their needs in a respectful yet direct way—no self-putdowns required.

HOW TO DO THE ACTIVITY ||||||||||||||||||||||||||||||||||||||||||||||||||||||||||||||||||

1. In the left column, write a list of phrases or words that you or other people say when they're feeling mad, sad, frustrated, embarrassed, or another big feeling. These phrases are usually negative. There are some examples to get you started.

2. In the column on the right side, write a list of alternate phrases or words that you could say to replace those you wrote in the left column. These phrases should still allow you to say what you mean, but in a way that is more positive than negative.

Negative phrases	Positive phrases
I can't do this.	*I'm still figuring this out.*
I shouldn't have done that.	*Here's what I learned when I did that.*
I'm so stupid.	*I'm learning.*
This is terrible.	*This is a challenge. I can handle it.*
I messed up.	*I can learn from this mistake.*
It's not fair.	*This isn't what I wanted.*

DESCRIBE YOUR GOLD STAR DAY

Our days don't always go exactly as planned. Sometimes we stub our toe, get a bad grade, or make a mistake during a game.

When we're going through big changes in our lives, like becoming part of a blended family, it's especially common to have "off" days. But for all the tough days you may have, you'll have plenty of wonderful days, too.

In this activity, you get to use your imagination and describe what a "Gold Star Day" would look like for you.

MATERIALS NEEDED

Pen or pencil

TIPS FOR PARENTS AND CAREGIVERS

This activity uses the power of visualization to help kids articulate what they enjoy and how they like to spend their time. I suggest going over your kids' Gold Star Day and then figuring out a way to make some (or even all) of this day a reality.

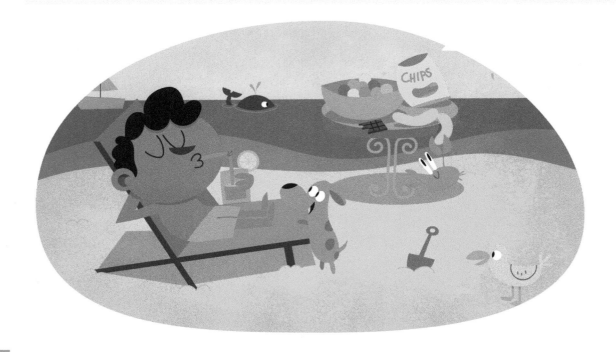

HOW TO DO THE ACTIVITY

1. Use your imagination to think about what your perfect day would look like from start to finish. If you can do anything you wanted, what would you do?

   - Where are you? Are you at home? Are you on a tropical island? Are you at a beach house? Are you in a new and exciting city?

   - What do you eat for breakfast?

   - What clothes do you put on? Do you have a favorite pair of jeans or shirt? Maybe you'd love a brand-new outfit. Imagine it!

   - What activities do you do throughout the day?

   - Who are you with?

   - What do you eat for dinner?

   - What time do you go to bed?

2. Remember, this is *your* Gold Star Day. It can be anything you want!

_____

_____

_____

_____

_____

_____

_____

_____

_____

25 HOW DO YOU LIKE TO SHOW LOVE?

Do you know there's more than one way to say, "I love you"?

You can show love by saying something nice, doing something kind or helpful, giving a gift, spending quality time together, or touching someone in a loving way.

Most of us like to show and be shown love in *all* these ways, but each of us usually has one or two ways that we like the most—and the way we like to receive love from others is usually the way we tend to show our love the most.

But a lot of times, the people around us like to be shown love in a way that's *different* from the way we like—it's as if we speak different languages.

When you know how your parent, sibling, or someone else you care about likes to receive love, you can show them how you feel by using *their* love language—even if it's not the same as yours. It's a great way to make sure everyone in your family feels loved and lovable.

MATERIALS NEEDED

Pens, pencils, or other coloring and drawing utensils

HOW TO DO THE ACTIVITY

1. On the first drawing page, use your imagination to write down or draw all your favorite ways to show love to your family members. Think of as many ideas as you can, like helping cook dinner, cuddling during a movie, giving a high five, doing chores around the house, reading together, or telling your family what makes them special.

2. On the second drawing page, use your imagination to write or draw all your favorite ways for your family to show their love for you. What's the most important to you? Think of ideas like going out to your favorite restaurant, receiving a surprise or a gift, hearing a nice compliment like "you are so talented!", getting a hug, or being picked up from school.

3. After both pages are full of your expressions of love, share them with your family members. Tell them what ways are most important to you and then ask what their favorites are too. Talk about how you can practice these in the future.

TIPS FOR PARENTS AND CAREGIVERS

The five love languages were first described in a 1992 book written by Gary Chapman. Understanding that people tend to show love in the way they prefer *to be shown* love is a powerful paradigm shift for relationships. Not only does it help your loved ones feel and notice *your* love, but it also helps you notice all the ways your loved ones show their love to *you*. I recommend writing down a list of each family member's top two or three love languages. Keep this in mind as you move forward and build connections with your blended family.

Continued ▶

HOW I LIKE TO BE LOVED

HOW I LIKE TO SHOW LOVE

WHICH FICTIONAL CHARACTER ARE YOU?

Think about your favorite character. Is this character from a Disney movie or a video game? Or maybe they're from a book you like to read or a television show you like to watch? Have you seen this character on YouTube or in a magazine?

It doesn't matter if this pretend character is a human, a dog, a fairy, a superhero, or any other creation. Whoever or whatever they are, you have a lot more in common with them than you think!

MATERIALS NEEDED

Drawing utensils, such as pens, pencils, colored pencils, or crayons

TIPS FOR PARENTS AND CAREGIVERS

I love the idea that the world is a mirror: *you can only see in others what you have in yourself.* This belief can keep you humble when you're feeling frustrated or annoyed by someone—but it also keeps you hopeful when someone inspires and motivates you.

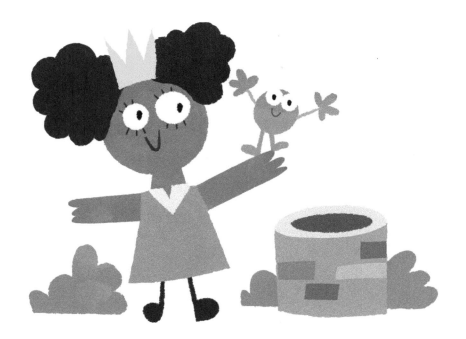

HOW TO DO THE ACTIVITY ||||||||||||||||||||||||||||||||||||||||||||||||||||||

1. On the left side of the drawing space, draw your favorite character. On the right side, draw a picture of yourself. Use whatever colors, designs, and shapes you'd like for both drawings.

2. Take some time to think about what it is you love about your favorite character. Are they brave, athletic, kind, thoughtful, or something else? Write down all these characteristics in the middle section.

3. Now look at the picture of yourself. Think of a time in your life when you showed each one of those characteristics that you love about your favorite character. Did you have any idea that the two of you were so similar?

My Favorite Character	What I Love about Them	Myself
	_____	
	_____	
	_____	
	_____	
	_____	
	_____	
	_____	
	_____	
	_____	
	_____	
	_____	
	_____	
	_____	
	_____	
	_____	

Have you noticed how good it feels to do nice things for other people?

When you bring a smile to other people's faces, it really helps put a smile on yours, too. That's because being generous and kind reminds you of the great person you are inside. And even when you're not feeling great, that great person is still there—and still able to help others.

In this activity, you get to spread some positivity around your home and share smiles with your family . . . just using some sticky notes. It's like sprinkling happiness all over your house!

MATERIALS NEEDED

Pens, markers, or colored pencils   Sticky notes

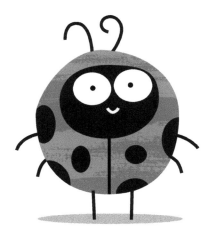

HOW TO DO THE ACTIVITY

1. Gather all your drawing tools and supplies.

2. Write down kind words and phrases on your sticky notes. Be as creative as you wish! Look at the examples on this page for inspiration.

3. Go around your home and post the sticky notes in different places. Consider some of these creative places to share some smiles:

   - The bathroom mirrors
   - Inside a cabinet or drawer
   - Under someone's pillow
   - Inside someone's coat pocket

Respect people's privacy, please! Be sure to ask your grown-ups for permission to hang your sticky notes, and make sure it's okay to go into your siblings' or parents' bedrooms before you do so.

You look great today! You are strong, brave, kind, and loving.	I love you.	I'm proud of you.
I'm thankful for you.	I'm so glad to be here with you.	Go ahead and smile!
Have a great day.	Just a reminder: you're awesome!	You can do it!
I like you.	I love playing games with you.	Thank you for being you!
You are a great cook.	I love your hugs.	Thinking about you!

What does it mean to have self-esteem?

Kids with self-esteem can feel proud of what they do. They like themselves, even when they make a mistake. Self-esteem is like a rocket ship that can help you go to some amazing places!

This activity helps you build your self-esteem so that you can do all the wonderful things you want in life with more confidence and love for yourself.

MATERIALS NEEDED

Pens, pencils, and other
  drawing utensils

Paper or cardstock
Kid-safe scissors

TIPS FOR PARENTS AND CAREGIVERS

We want our children to understand how building their self-esteem will help them see the good in themselves, in other people, and in other things. Self-esteem can also help them weather the most challenging and scary moments in their lives. We must "fill our own tanks" with self-directed goodness and care if we want to get out there and enjoy life.

HOW TO DO THE ACTIVITY

1. Use your imagination to draw a rocket ship on your piece of paper. When you're done, carefully cut out your rocket ship using scissors.

2. Your rocket ship isn't ready to blast off to outer space just yet—it needs fuel! We're going to fuel your rocket ship with self-esteem. Next to each number in the table on this page, write down something you're good at, something you like about yourself, or something you've achieved.

3. Once you have made your list of 10 things, your rocket ship's fuel tank is full and ready to go. Read aloud each item one at a time, like you're doing a countdown. Then . . . blastoff! It's time to run around and play with your rocket ship!

Rocket fuel: What are you good at? What do you like about yourself?	
10.	
9.	
8.	
7.	
6.	
5.	
4.	
3.	
2.	
1.	

_____ AND THE TERRIBLE, HORRIBLE, NO GOOD, VERY BAD DAY

When your family is changing, it's normal to have days when everything just seems turned upside down. Maybe you can think of a day when you felt totally unloved, as if nobody liked you or even noticed you.

MATERIALS NEEDED

2 different colored pens or pencils

TIPS FOR PARENTS AND CAREGIVERS

Do you remember this book from when you were a child? *Alexander and the Terrible, Horrible, No Good, Very Bad Day* is a classic children's book written in 1972 by Judith Viorst and illustrated by Ray Cruz. Grab yourself a copy and read it with the whole family!

You might find it strange to have your kids write in detail about a day that went, in their estimation, totally wrong. However, research shows that when we write about stressful or challenging events, it can help us process our emotions better, and we can learn valuable lessons from these events, too.

HOW TO DO THE ACTIVITY

1. Think about a recent day you had when some things, many things, or maybe *everything* just seemed to go wrong.

2. Using one pen, describe this day like you're telling a story. Detail each thing that happened that made you feel bad.

3. Once you've written about your tough day in as much detail as possible, go back and reread it. Do any feelings come up inside your body as you do this?

4. Next use your imagination to think about how you could have done things differently if you had to live that day over again. What could you have done (or not done) that would have helped you feel safer, calmer, or less upset? What did you learn from this day? Use your other pen to write down your ideas.

_____ and the Terrible, Horrible, No Good, Very Bad Day

How Things Could Have Gone Differently

30 MAKING MY "FEEL GOOD" COLLAGE

The beauty of being in a blended family is that different personalities get to come together and create an interesting and colorful household.

In addition to leaning on each other for support, you can also create your own little moments of peace and calm. In this activity, you'll create a piece of art that you can look at whenever you need a little extra help to feel good.

|||||||||||||||||||||||||||||||||||||||||| MATERIALS NEEDED ||||||||||||||||||||||||||||||

Pens, pencils, and other
  drawing utensils
Old magazines

Kid-safe scissors
Glue

HOW TO DO THE ACTIVITY

1. Gather your drawing utensils and supplies.

2. Cut out images, words, and colors from old magazines. Look for things that stand out to you—things that you find interesting, cool, pretty, calming, or just awesome. When you look at the images you've cut out, notice how you feel. If you feel good when you look at them, then they are perfect for you!

3. Take your magazine clippings and glue them to the blank space on page 72. This is called a *collage*: sticking or gluing different pieces of paper or other materials together to form one larger art piece.

4. Add whatever else you'd like to your collage. Take your time, and don't stop until you feel like you've made a piece of art that you love looking at. It doesn't have to be perfect, just filled with images, colors, and words that bring a smile to your face.

The next time you're feeling worried, stressed, or upset, see what happens when you look at your collage quietly for a few minutes as you take slow, deep breaths. Notice if you feel any better after spending some time in front of your own art.

TIPS FOR PARENTS AND CAREGIVERS

Creativity is one of the best avenues we have for processing difficult emotions. In this creative activity, your kids get to spend time immersed in images and words that bring them joy—and they also have a piece of art that they can hold on to and look at later. Seeing how unique each of your kids' collages is can be a great reminder of how they see the world through completely different lenses. Understanding this is a good way to support them through important life transitions.

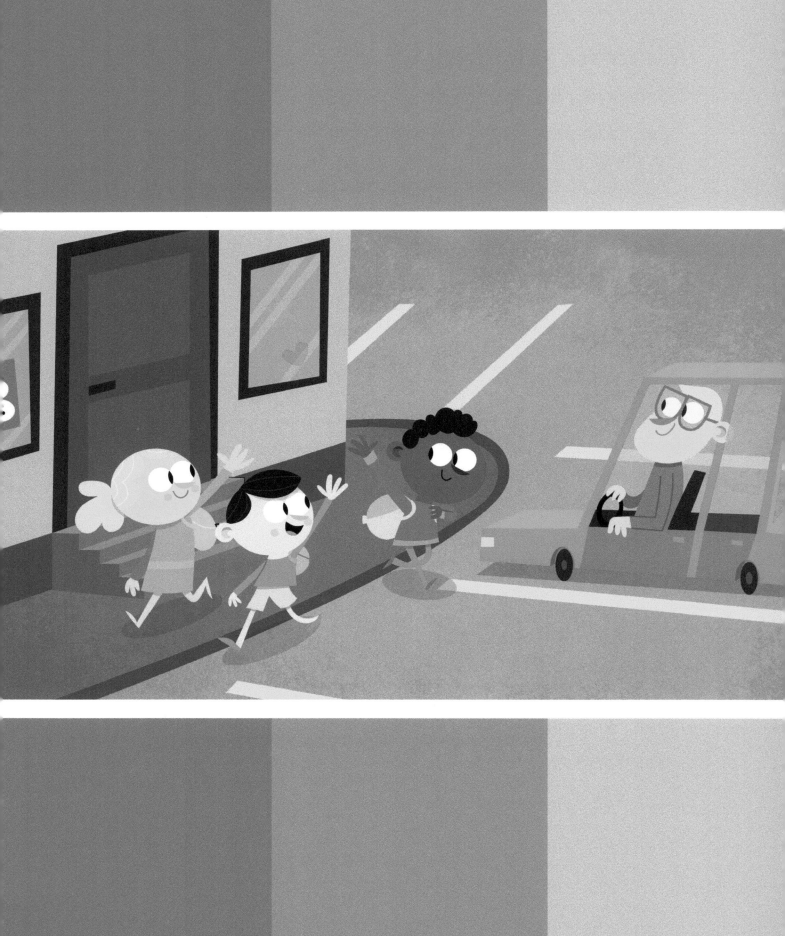

CHAPTER 4

I Can Learn and Grow through New Relationships

Tom and his friends Jen and Kevin are waiting outside the school during afternoon pickup. Tom sees his caregiver drive up to the pickup line. Tom waves, then grabs his backpack.

He turns to his friends and says, "See you guys tomorrow!"

As Tom walks away, Jen looks confused. "Who is that?" she asks, pointing at the man driving the car that Tom gets into. "That's not his dad."

"That's Tom's stepdad," Kevin says. "He's married to Tom's mom."

"Oh," Jen says. She thinks for a moment, then says, "Well, isn't Tom's mom supposed to be married to Tom's dad?"

Kevin sees his own mom drive up to the pickup line. "Not all parents are like that," he says, slinging his backpack over his shoulder. "My mom told me that sometimes different families grow and change."

"Does Tom still have a dad?" she asks.

"Yeah," Kevin says. "I saw him at our little league game last week."

Jen thinks about this. "Wow," she says. "Tom has more than two parents. Cool!"

INTRODUCTION

When you become a part of a blended family, you probably get to meet a lot of new people. You get to start building and exploring many new relationships. How fun! Just think of all the people who might be in your life now:

- Stepparents

- Stepsiblings

- New extended family members, including your stepsiblings' grandparents, aunts, uncles, and cousins

- New family friends

- Maybe even some new family pets!

No matter how many new relationships and family members you have now, it's important to remember that you *belong* in your growing family. It's safe for you to be who you are, even when there are so many new people to get to know.

And, yes, I know the process of starting a family with new people can be a little scary at times. Other members of your blended family might even be a little nervous, too! That's why working together to get to know each other and build trust is so helpful. It helps your new family start to feel like a team that works together to feel happy, safe, and loved.

By the way . . .

Even though you have a whole new group of family members to get to know, nobody can replace your biological parents and siblings ("biological" means the family you were born into). Your relationships with your parents and siblings won't go away just because you're building new relationships with new family members.

In fact, the activities in this chapter—which are meant to help you and your blended family members get closer and have fun together—are great to do with your biological family members, too. The more the merrier!

Let's get started.

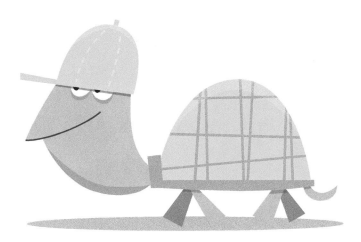

GUESS WHO? BLENDED FAMILY EDITION

Playing board games is a great way to spend time with your new family and get to know each other. One of my favorite games to play growing up was Guess Who?

In this activity, you try to guess who is on your opponent's Mystery card—before they guess who is on yours. The twist is that you'll add photos of your own family members into the mix. This "family edition" of Guess Who? is a really fun way to get to know your new family members and identify some of the things that make each of you special and unique.

|||||||||||||||||||||||||||||||||||| MATERIALS NEEDED ||||||||||||||||||||||||||||||||||||

The Guess Who? board game
3 small photos of each of your family members (or photos that can be cut to size)

Kid-safe scissors
Tape

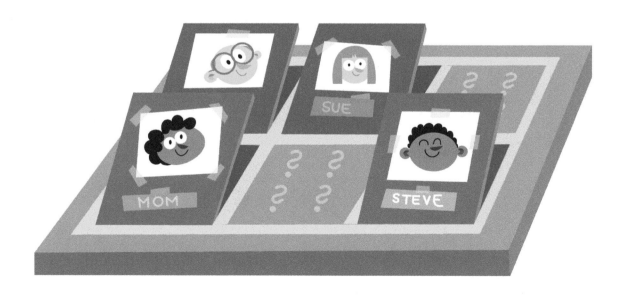

HOW TO DO THE ACTIVITY

1. Gather your supplies and take out the Guess Who? game.

2. Insert one small picture of each of your family members into the red and blue trays. (Your parents or caregivers can help you cut the photos to the right size so they'll fit.) Use the game's original cards for any of the remaining spaces—there are 40 on each board.

3. Tape the other small picture of each of your family members onto a Mystery card. Make sure any remaining original cards have a match on the red and blue trays.

4. Shuffle the deck of Mystery cards. Each person draws a card and places the card facing them into the slot on their tray. Make sure you can't see each other's cards!

5. The first player asks a question about their opponent's Mystery Person. All questions must be answered with a yes or a no.

   Example: "Does your Mystery Person have blue eyes?" If the answer is yes, look carefully at all the people on your tray and eliminate (flip down) anyone who doesn't have blue eyes. If the answer is no, you can eliminate anyone who has blue eyes.

6. Keep taking turns asking your yes/no questions until someone thinks they're ready to guess who is on their opponent's Mystery card. It could be a family member or an original character from the game. Either way, it's super fun!

TIPS FOR PARENTS AND CAREGIVERS

Guess Who? is intended for only two players, so take turns. While playing this game, help your kids get creative about their questions. It's fine to ask about physical characteristics, such as eye color, skin color, and so on. They can also ask other types of questions that will help them get to know different family members—from whether they speak multiple languages or use any adaptive equipment to what their job, favorite hobby, or favorite color is.

Think about your new family. Even though you all have many differences, you're still connected. This is just one thing that makes your new family so great.

After all, when multiple people come together and form new connections, they can build something strong and durable—kind of like a spider web.

Have you ever seen a spider web before? It might look fragile, but scientists believe that if a spider web was human-size, it would be strong enough to trap an airplane—wow! This activity is a chance to see some of the connections you're building with your new family and help you realize how strong these connections can be.

MATERIALS NEEDED

A large ball of string

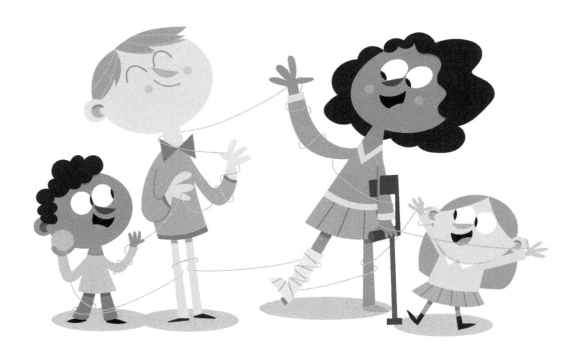

HOW TO DO THE ACTIVITY

1. Get all your family members together and stand in a large circle.

2. Give the ball of string to one person in the circle. Have this person say something they really like, such as "I like playing outside," or "I love dogs." They may also choose to say something they *don't* like, such as "I don't like cantaloupe," or "I don't like scary movies."

3. Anyone else in the circle who likes (or dislikes) the same thing should raise their hand. The person holding the string looks around the circle for someone raising their hand and then hands the ball of string to that person while holding the end of the string in their own hand.

4. Now the next person holding the ball of string says something they like or dislike. Anyone who agrees raises their hand, and the person passes the ball of string along while still holding on to a bit of string in their hand.

5. Keep repeating this until the ball of string has been passed around to everyone at least 3 times.

Pretty soon, you'll see a huge web forming within the circle. Notice the size, shape, and pattern of the web you're making together! Feel free to pull, tug, and twist a little and see just how strong the connections really are.

TIPS FOR PARENTS AND CAREGIVERS

This web-making game helps your kids recognize all the similarities and differences within their new family. It's a fun way to make connections and have those "Hey, me, too!" moments.

If you don't have a large ball of string handy, you can try doing this activity outside on the pavement with some chalk. Simply draw your web on the ground, and watch it grow.

33 TWO TRUTHS AND A MAKE-BELIEVE

Two Truths and a Make-Believe is a fun game that requires no special supplies. You can even do this game during a long car ride or while out on a family hike.

In this game, you get to have fun trying to "trick" your family members . . . and they get to have fun trying to "trick" you! Along the way, you'll use your imagination and get to know interesting facts about your family members as well.

MATERIALS NEEDED

Pen or pencil

TIPS FOR PARENTS AND CAREGIVERS

You can play this game just for fun, or you can keep score. If you're keeping score, the person making statements gets a point if the other family members can't correctly guess the pretend answer.

This is a fun and creative way to learn interesting facts about your new family members. You may be surprised by what you'll find out!

HOW TO DO THE ACTIVITY

1. Get together with your family. One person makes three statements about themselves. Two of these statements must be true, and one must be pretend or make-believe.

2. Everyone else in the family has to try to guess which statement is the make-believe one.

The goal is to trick people into thinking that one of your *true* statements is actually make-believe. To do this, it helps to make your make-believe statement sound believable or almost real. For instance, you might say:

I got three stitches when I was five.

I can play the piano.

I've never seen the movie *Frozen*.

All of these statements sound like they could be true. Unless your family members really know you, they might have a hard time figuring out which one is pretend.

1. _____ 2. _____ 3. _____	1. _____ 2. _____ 3. _____	1. _____ 2. _____ 3. _____
1. _____ 2. _____ 3. _____	1. _____ 2. _____ 3. _____	1. _____ 2. _____ 3. _____

Getting to know your blended family can feel like a roller-coaster ride. Some days, you might feel excited, happy, and glad about the changes going on in your home. On other days, you might feel scared, sad, lonely, or angry. It's totally normal to have your feelings go up and down.

Don't forget that other people in your family might have up-and-down feelings, too. But the goal isn't for everyone to feel good all the time—it's for everyone in your family to express their feelings in a way that doesn't hurt themselves or other people.

This weeklong family photo challenge is a good place to start!

MATERIALS NEEDED

Your phone's camera and self-timer feature

Pen or pencil

TIPS FOR PARENTS AND CAREGIVERS

If you can, I recommend getting together for your daily portrait at the same time each day. As you sit down with your kids and look through all the pictures, ask guiding questions that will help them notice and become curious about their siblings' and stepsiblings' feelings. They might ask things like:

- You look angry in this picture. Were you feeling angry that day?
- Do you remember why you were feeling happy/sad/angry that day?

HOW TO DO THE ACTIVITY

1. Get together with your family. It's great to start this activity on a Monday, but any day of the week will do.

2. Everyone takes 1 minute to think about how they are feeling at that particular moment.

3. Next think about how you might show other people what you're feeling using a particular pose or facial expression. Are you feeling happy and want to smile or jump? Are you feeling angry and want to scrunch your eyebrows together?

4. Now stand in front of the camera and take a family photo. Everyone should be posing in a way that reflects how they feel at that moment.

5. Meet up every day for the next 5 days to do the same thing.

6. After 5 days, sit down as a family and go through all the photos. Use the chart on this page to record how everyone's feelings can change throughout the week!

Day 1	Day 2	Day 3	Day 4	Day 5
_____	_____	_____	_____	_____
_____	_____	_____	_____	_____
_____	_____	_____	_____	_____
_____	_____	_____	_____	_____
_____	_____	_____	_____	_____

Trusting people you're still getting to know can be scary. But sometimes the best way to start building trust in someone is to be brave and show them that they can trust you!

This activity is a fun and exciting way to help you and your new family members learn how to depend on each other. Trust falls show how you will be there to support each other during this big transition in your life.

MATERIALS NEEDED

An open space, ideally with a soft surface (like carpet or grass)

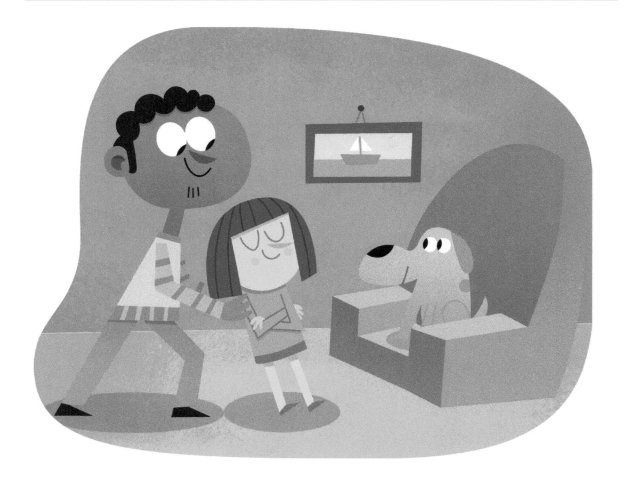

HOW TO DO THE ACTIVITY

1. Pair up with one of your family members, and stand, if you are able to, facing each other.

2. One person in the pair then turns around, facing away from their partner. The person who turns around is the "faller." They will keep their arms crossed on their chest, legs stiff, and feet together.

3. The "catcher" should get into the following position: one leg back and straight, one leg forward and bent, and both arms slightly bent in front of the chest with palms facing toward the faller's back.

4. Use verbal cues to prepare for the fall:

   - Faller says, "Spotter ready?"
   - Catcher says, "Ready."
   - Faller says, "Falling."
   - Catcher says, "Fall away."

5. The faller leans back and starts to fall. Using their hands and body, the catcher will gently catch the person and help them back to the starting position.

6. After doing this once, switch roles so the catcher gets to be the faller and vice versa.

You can repeat the exercise a few times and then try with someone else in the family.

TIPS FOR PARENTS AND CAREGIVERS

Safety, safety, safety! Be sure to practice the verbal cues and falling and catching positions with your family *before* starting this activity.

Also keep in mind that different family members have different bodies. Provide backup support to anyone who might need it. You may also choose to modify the fall to make sure all your kids stay comfortable, depending on their mobility—for instance, you can try this sitting on the floor.

Do you love listening to stories? How about telling stories?

The truth is, storytelling is a great way to bond with other people. Creating stories as a family can bring you closer together, and it helps you share things you've learned from your own life experiences. After all, everyone you meet has something interesting to say . . . and when you listen, you might even learn something useful!

MATERIALS NEEDED

Sticky notes or index cards
Pen

Tape

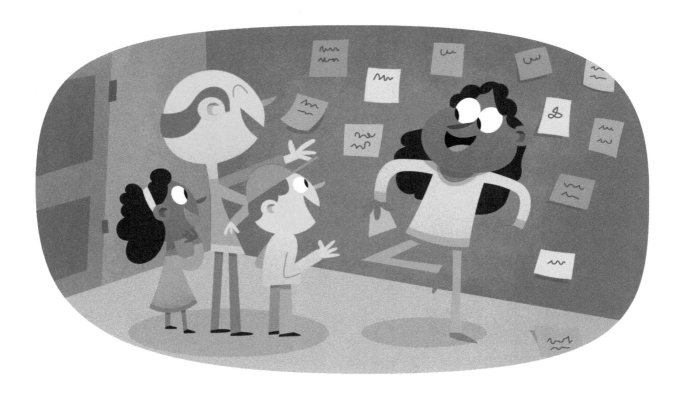

HOW TO DO THE ACTIVITY IIIIIIIIIIIIIIIIIIIIIIIIIIIIIIIIIIIIIIIIIIIIIIIIIIIIIIIIIIIIIIIIIIIIIIIIIIII

1. Sit down with your family. Work together to come up with 10 to 20 words or phrases you can use as special words to start the storytelling session. Write each word on a sticky note or index card. These should be positive words that remind you of good things for you and your new family members. Try words such as *trust, friendship, teamwork, loyalty, safety, belonging, brave,* and *fun*.

2. Post the sticky notes on a nearby wall where everyone can see them.

3. Have everyone look at the sticky notes for about 1 to 3 minutes and think of a story or memory associated with one of the words.

4. Have someone go first by picking a sticky note with their chosen word on it and moving it to a blank spot on the wall. Then they tell a story that the word made them think of.

5. The next person will peel another word from the wall and post it next to the word put up by the first person. This is the start of a "story thread." The person then tells their story.

6. Make sure everyone listens closely as the stories are being told. If a person's story reminds you of a new word, you can jot this down on a new sticky note and put it up when it's your turn. Otherwise, you can pull a sticky note from the original group.

7. Repeat this process until the players have created a snakelike story thread. Look at all the ways your conversation twisted and turned!

TIPS FOR PARENTS AND CAREGIVERS

You can decide as a family when the storytelling ends or give a specific time limit. Before you "put out" the campfire and take down the sticky notes, be sure to ask your family members if they have any final thoughts or things on their mind.

FAMILY TIME ON TIKTOK!

Have you heard of TikTok?

This social media app is a fun way to try out funny scenes, dances, and challenges. Doing TikTok challenges together is also a great way to bond when you're hanging out at home and getting to know each other as a family.

Another great thing about TikTok challenges is that you can record them. You'll have funny videos to look back at together, and you can also share them with friends and other family members.

This activity describes one popular dance known as the "Something New Challenge."

MATERIALS NEEDED

Internet-accessible phone with a camera

TikTok app

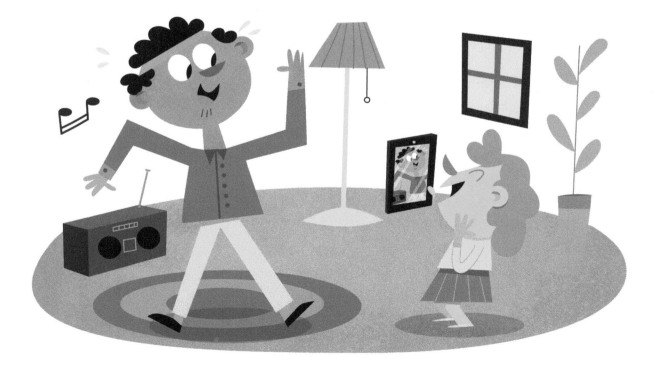

HOW TO DO THE ACTIVITY |||||||||||||||||||||||||||||||||||||||||||||||||||||||||||||||||||||||||||||||||||

1. Have everyone in the family stand in a line, one behind the other, with the first person facing the camera.

2. Play the song "Something New" from the TikTok app.

3. Keeping in time with the music, have the first person do a little dance move, then jump out of the line and out of the camera's view.

4. The next person in line does a little dance move, then they jump out of the line.

5. Keep going until everyone in the family has had their moment to wiggle in front of the camera!

TIPS FOR PARENTS AND CAREGIVERS

There are tons of different TikTok challenges and dances. The "Something New Challenge" is a great way to "introduce" your entire family. Each person gets their moment in the spotlight and can move their body however they see fit!

If you're not a fan of TikTok or this song in particular, feel free to do a DIY version of this dance challenge with your phone camera and a song that's a family favorite.

Cooking at home with whole ingredients—like veggies, fruits, grains, meat, chicken, fish, spices, and sauces—is so good for your body! Plus, it's fun to see all the ingredients come together in a delicious and nutritious meal.

Cooking for your family is also a great way to show them you care. That's why this activity allows everyone in your family to take turns being the "chef for the day." (A chef is someone whose job is to cook.)

Look forward to a week of interesting new dishes to try. Keep in mind that some dishes might be a lot different from what you're used to eating. Do your best to keep an open mind and be willing to try new things. You never know what you might like!

MATERIALS NEEDED

A cookbook or favorite recipe   Ingredients

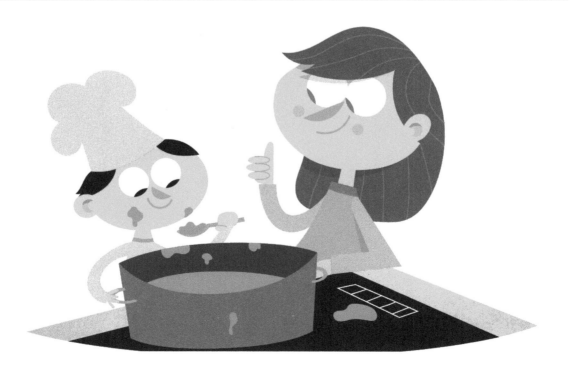

HOW TO DO THE ACTIVITY

1. Assign each person in your family a night to cook. Then have each person think of a recipe they want to make for dinner. This could be a recipe for a totally new meal or a longtime favorite dish.

2. Take your recipes and head to the grocery store. Gather all the ingredients you'll need.

3. Each night, sit down together as a group, and enjoy the meal cooked by one of your family members. You can make it extra fun by adding some table decorations, dressing up, or making special themes.

4. Be sure to take turns helping to clean up, too.

TIPS FOR PARENTS AND CAREGIVERS

Let's face it: food is a *huge* part of family time. When families come together with different cultures, preferences, and traditions, the impact on mealtime can be quite noticeable. This may be hard on your kids if they're picky about what they eat, are missing a favorite meal or snack, or are simply still adjusting to the changes going on in your family.

Getting kids involved in the kitchen is a perfect way to help them feel more in control. This benefits their decision-making skills and creativity, and also gives them a great sense of accomplishment and confidence when they see everyone sitting down and eating the food they cooked.

Be sure to provide whatever supervision is necessary for your kids depending on their age and abilities. As always, take any food allergies or sensitivities into consideration.

39 FINDING THE SILVER LINING

Being a part of a family means that you have many shared memories of things you've done together. But not everyone in a family remembers past events in the exact same way, especially if the events were negative, scary, or tough. And this doesn't mean that one person's memory is necessarily "wrong" and another person's memory is "right"—it's just that different people often have different ways of looking at things.

In this activity, you'll sit down as a family and talk about some tough moments from your past. You'll get a chance to practice good listening skills and even help each other learn to see the "silver lining."

A silver lining is like finding a positive in a negative or a good thing that happened during or even because of a bad experience. Once we learn to look for the silver linings in even our toughest, scariest moments, we can start to change our points of view and feel more hopeful and excited about our future.

MATERIALS NEEDED

Pen or pencil

_____

_____

_____

_____

_____

_____

HOW TO DO THE ACTIVITY

1. Ask everyone in your family to spend about 5 minutes thinking about a challenging memory or tough moment from the past and write down a few notes about it. This memory could involve other people in the family, people at school, or something else altogether. Write down anything that comes to mind. If it helps, think about a time when you were sad, scared, mad, frustrated, bored, or lonely, or when something unexpected happened.

2. Take turns reading aloud what you've written down.

3. After someone is done telling their story, have everyone else in the group brainstorm about possible silver linings that they see in their story. The person who told their own story can help, too.

Here's an example:

Sarah tells a story about how one time she was embarrassed that her teacher called her stepmom her mom in front of all her friends. Her stepsiblings put their heads together and helped Sarah find the following silver linings:

- *Sarah got to practice speaking up for herself.*

- *Her teacher now knows who Sarah's stepmom is, so she won't make that mistake again.*

- *Sarah learned that her friends don't care if her parents are divorced—in fact, Sarah found out that some of her friends' parents are divorced, too.*

TIPS FOR PARENTS AND CAREGIVERS

Sometimes it's hard to find the silver lining in our toughest moments. The goal of this activity is not to negate or belittle someone's experience, but simply to invite them to shift their perspective on it and see it in a different light.

A motto is a short phrase or sentence that describes the shared beliefs, ideas, and goals of a person or group of people.

Mottos are useful because they:

* Remind us of how we want to live our lives and what kind of people we want to be

* Remind us of the kinds of qualities or characteristics we want to strengthen and improve in ourselves

* Help us set goals and take actions that will help us achieve these goals

Did you know your family can have its very own motto, too? In this activity, you get to use your creativity to come up with a special saying that your new blended family can use as daily inspiration.

MATERIALS NEEDED

Drawing utensils and any other art supplies you want

A large piece of poster board or cardstock

HOW TO DO THE ACTIVITY

1. Get together as a family and gather all your drawing supplies.

2. Spend at least 10 to 20 minutes coming up with ideas for a family motto. Be as creative as you'd like! If it helps, think about what sorts of things your family finds important, like happiness, trust, kindness, respect, and inclusion. Here are some examples to get you started:

   - The Martinez-Jones Family: Strong, Safe, and Smiling

   - The Peterson Family: Happy, Humble, Honest, and Kind

   - The Lee Family: Working Together to Make Today the Best Day!

   - The Johnson-Young Team: Taking Care of Our Health, Our Minds, Our Home, Our Planet, and Each Other

   - The Rodgers Family: We Show Respect with Our Words and Actions

3. Once you've agreed on your family motto, write it in big letters on a piece of sturdy paper. Decorate the paper using markers, colored pencils, and any other materials you'd like.

Hang your completed poster somewhere in your home where you all can see your motto and think about it often: on the fridge, in the mudroom, or in a main hallway are all great places.

TIPS FOR PARENTS AND CAREGIVERS

Coming up with a motto is a great way for kids to build a sense of connection, cohesion, and clarity in their new family. When you start this activity together, start from the gold standard perspective of a true brainstorming session: *all* ideas are welcome and worth writing down. Learning how to work together, make compromises, and listen to new ideas is a valuable skill for everyone in your family to hone during this major transition.

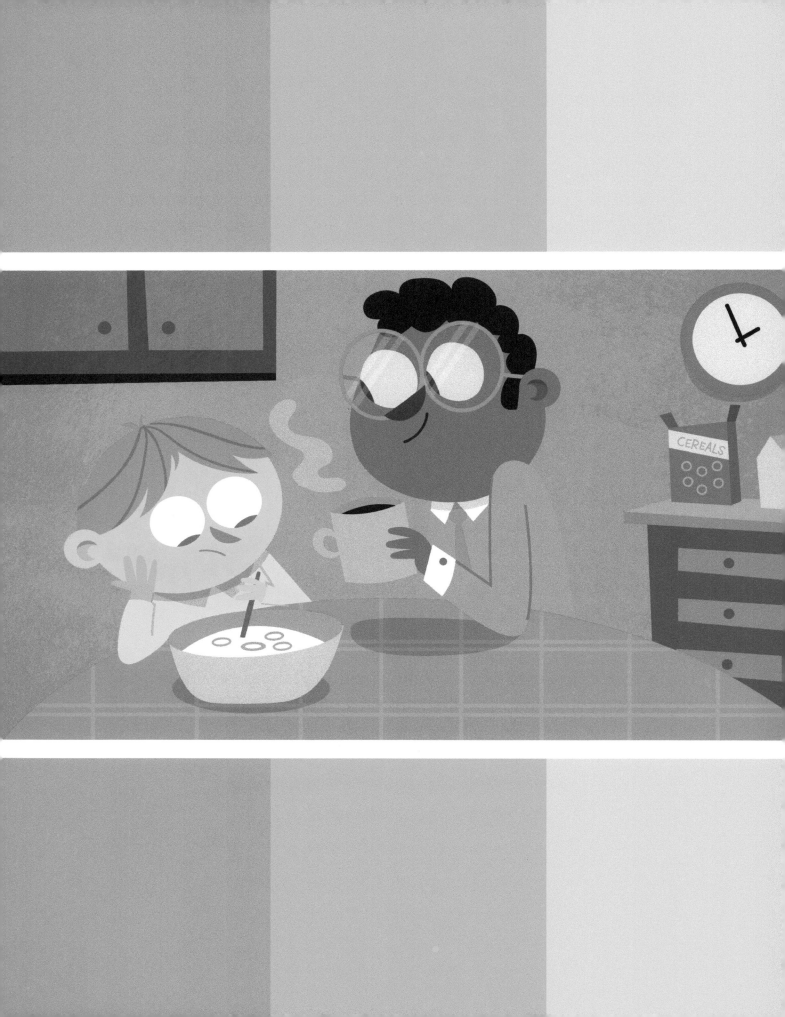

CHAPTER 5

Speaking Up for Myself Makes Everyone Feel Better

Stomp. Stomp. Stomp. Jeremiah plods down the stairs and walks into the kitchen. He sits down at the table in a huff and immediately places his head in his hands.

Jeremiah's stepdad walks over to him and places a bowl of oatmeal in front of him. "Good morning, Jeremiah," he says.

Jeremiah grumbles in response.

His stepdad sits down at the table next to him. "If there's anything you want to tell me, if there's anything on your mind, I'm here and ready to listen," he says. Then he takes a sip of his coffee.

Jeremiah looks up at his stepdad. He sighs and then starts poking at his oatmeal with a spoon. "I could barely sleep all night because I could hear my stepbrother snoring from his room. I'm so annoyed!"

His stepdad nods. "I can see how that would be frustrating. I'm sorry you had to deal with that last night." He thinks for a moment, taking a slow sip of his coffee. "Do you think it would help if we bought you a fan or a white noise machine for your room?"

"Yeah!" Jeremiah says, perking up. "I think it would!"

INTRODUCTION

Did you know there's something about you that *nobody* else has?

Okay, there are actually a *lot* of things about you that nobody else has. But the best thing you have that no one else does is your *voice*.

What you think, how you feel, and how you choose to express yourself are all a part of your unique voice. You use your voice to ask for what you need, communicate what you're thinking and feeling, and stand up for yourself (or others) when it's time to stand up. You can even use your voice to help others feel better!

That's why the people in your life who love and care about you want to hear what you have to say. But how can we use our voice clearly to tell others what we need, even when we're feeling uncomfortable or going through a tough time?

This chapter is dedicated to helping you learn how to do just that. The activities that follow can help you:

- Practice your communication skills

- Try different ways to express yourself—both verbally (with words) and nonverbally (with your body and the tone of your voice)

- Learn how to be true to yourself, even when you need to say something that is uncomfortable

- See that it's safe to express your thoughts and feelings with your family

- Experience how saying how you feel can actually help other people too!

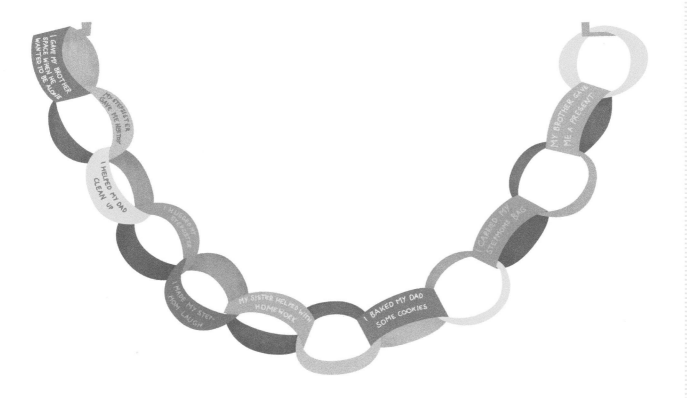

41 LIGHTS, CAMERA, ACTION!

Do you love to act or put on plays? In this fun activity, you get to learn and create through your imagination! Here's why this can help:

Pretending to act out a difficult conversation or situation ahead of time can help you feel braver if that actual conversation or situation comes up in your life. It's just like how actors rehearse (repeat and memorize) their lines before opening night: the more they practice, the better prepared they'll be for the real thing.

MATERIALS NEEDED

Clothing, props, and other
  materials for costumes (optional)
Index cards

Pen or pencil
Space for a "stage"

Someone is sad because they miss a parent who doesn't live with them.	Someone is having a hard time adjusting to a new rule in the household, especially if it's different at their other parent's house.	Someone wants to borrow their stepsibling's toy.	Someone at school mistakenly called a kid's stepparent their parent.	Someone is hogging the bathroom.
Someone is sad they missed a group outing because they were at their other parent's house.	_____ _____ _____ _____ _____ _____	_____ _____ _____ _____ _____ _____	_____ _____ _____ _____ _____ _____	_____ _____ _____ _____ _____ _____

HOW TO DO THE ACTIVITY

1. Sit down with your family. Working together, think of some tricky situations that might come up at home. You can include situations that have already come up for your blended family. Try to come up with at least 8 situations, and write each one down on an index card. Use the chart for some ideas or to brainstorm.

2. Now it's time to put on a show! Everyone takes a turn picking an index card and acting out the situation described. Try to think about how you would feel and all the different ways you can *show* someone how you're feeling instead of just saying it. Feel free to invite one of your family members up on your "stage" with you to act out the scene. You can take the lead, but act it out together.

3. When you're done with your scene, let people in the audience offer their ideas on different ways you could approach this situation.

TIPS FOR PARENTS AND CAREGIVERS

Giving your children a prompt and then allowing them to improvise and act out how they would respond to that situation is a great way to help them become more expressive and thoughtful about their feelings. Just think about it: How many times have you rehearsed a difficult conversation in your head?

42 EGG RACE

Body language is a form of communication, and it can say a lot! We use body language when we:

- Stand, sit, or position ourselves as tall or small

- Move our arms and hands

- Smile, frown, or grimace

- Jump, skip, dance, or stomp

In this activity, you get to experience using just body language to communicate with your family as you work together to accomplish a goal.

MATERIALS NEEDED

Spoons
Hard-boiled eggs

A clock (to keep track of time)

HOW TO DO THE ACTIVITY

1. As a family, create an obstacle course in your home (or backyard if you have one). The course should be made of items that people can move around, over, or under—whatever ways you like to use your bodies! Use the drawing space on page 104 to plan out your course first.

2. Pair up with a family member. Each pair should have two spoons and one egg.

3. One person in each pair begins by holding their spoon while balancing the egg on it.

4. As a team (pair), move through the obstacle course. Throughout the obstacle course, stop and pass the egg to each other, only using your spoons. You can have someone call out "Switch!" every 10 to 30 seconds, or you can pass the egg each time you complete one lap of the obstacle course.

Here's the real trick of the obstacle course: *No talking allowed!* You can use gestures or facial expressions to show your excitement and help each other get over obstacles, but you must not use words. See how far you can get without dropping your egg!

TIPS FOR PARENTS AND CAREGIVERS

This activity is a fun way for your kids to work together, and it's also an opportunity for them to step into their bodies a bit more and use body language to communicate how they're feeling. I recommend using hard-boiled eggs to avoid making a huge mess!

I've found that this activity can be done in small and large spaces. Get creative with how you design your obstacle courses to really challenge each other.

Isn't it interesting how two people can go through the same experience but have completely different perspectives and memories about it?

This doesn't mean one person is "right" and one person is "wrong." It just means that we have different eyes, different brains, and different hearts. This kind of variety is partially what makes it so interesting to make friends—or join a blended family. Coming together to celebrate what makes us unique helps make life interesting!

In this activity, you and your family members get to reflect on recent experiences together and share your unique perspectives, including the emotions you felt. Pay attention to how your emotions and memories are similar or different.

MATERIALS NEEDED

Space to sit together

HOW TO DO THE ACTIVITY

1. Get together as a family and sit in a circle.

2. Choose one person to sit in the middle of the circle. This person is the "thinker." Only the thinker has permission to talk. The job for everyone else in the circle is to listen.

3. The person in the middle starts the activity by saying, "I'm thinking of that time when . . ." Describe a situation that someone (or everyone) in the group recently experienced—maybe a trip to a restaurant or the mall, a party, a hike, or even a family meal together from the night before.

4. After the thinker describes how they felt during this situation and shares what they want to, they point to someone else in the circle and trade places with that person. The new person now sits in the middle and gets to share what they remember about the situation and how they felt.

5. Choose new thinkers to enter the circle and share their thoughts about the situation until everyone has said what they want to say.

TIPS FOR PARENTS AND CAREGIVERS

One of the best things you can do for your family is show they are safe to share how they think and feel about shared experiences—even if it's different from how other people think and feel.

The physical act of moving into the center of the circle to express your thoughts and feelings might feel a bit scary, as if you're delivering a public speech. But this can be a valuable exercise for helping your kids learn how to deal with the possible discomfort of speaking their minds.

Model to your children what it means to listen attentively and to offer empathy. Also, consider that any memory or shared experience can work well here—whether it's positive or negative.

44 | IT'S KARAOKE TIME!

Do you have a favorite song?

Maybe you know a song that reminds you of a special moment, place, or person. Perhaps you know a song that matches your personality or describes a situation that reminds you of what you're going through right now.

Music is such a gift to this world. It helps us tell stories, communicate with others, and move our bodies. In this activity, you and your family get to put on a karaoke night and sing the songs that you love together! (Karaoke is the activity where someone sings along to music.)

MATERIALS NEEDED

Space to sing and dance
A microphone (a pretend
   microphone works, too!)

A stereo or anything else that
   plays music
Pen or pencil

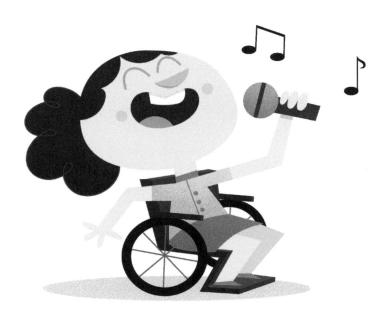

HOW TO DO THE ACTIVITY

1. Have each person in your family come up with a favorite song.

2. Using an app like Spotify or a website like YouTube, put all these songs in a playlist.

3. Choose one night this week to be Family Karaoke Night. Take turns singing your hearts out to your favorite tunes!

4. After each person gets a chance to sing their song, give them time to talk about why they like this song so much.

TIPS FOR PARENTS AND CAREGIVERS

Sometimes music has a way of expressing how we feel, even when we can't find the words ourselves. Creating a playlist encourages collaboration between your family members, and choosing a song encourages each person to get in touch with what they're feeling in a fun and creative way.

If you or any of your kids don't love singing, you can always have a family dance party instead that includes your favorite songs. Or you could listen to the family playlist while eating dinner together or going for a hike outside.

Just be sure to have time at the end of every song for each person to explain why they chose that song for the family playlist.

Family Member	Song	What It Means to Them

A FAMILY JOURNAL CHALLENGE

When we leave big feelings stuck inside us, they can make our bodies and our minds start to feel bad. The best thing you can do when you're feeling strong emotions is to tell someone what you're feeling. Even if it feels a bit scary, telling someone you trust about how you feel can get you the help you need and show you that it's safe to express yourself.

But what happens if you're just not ready to tell someone your big feelings? Good news: just writing down how you feel and what you think on a piece of paper can help!

MATERIALS NEEDED

Journals

Pens, pencils, or other coloring and drawing utensils

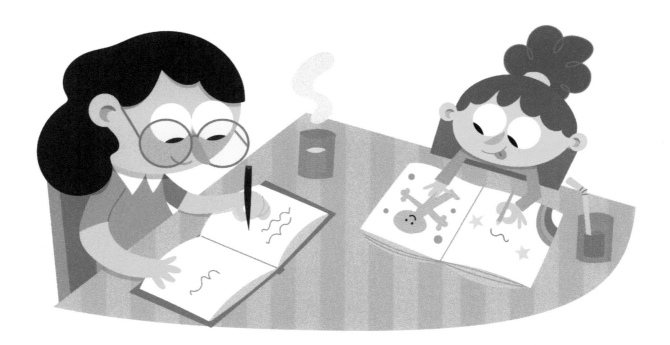

HOW TO DO THE ACTIVITY

1. Have everyone in the family create their own journal. Be creative! You can buy actual journals or make your own by stapling several pieces of paper together. Be sure to decorate your journal however you'd like. Make it your own!

2. As a family, choose a week that you'll all sit down at the same time each day and write in your journals for at least 5 minutes. Many families choose to do this Monday through Friday, right after breakfast or dinner. The cool thing about this is that even if some of you are in different houses at some point during the week, you can all write in your journals at the same time. So you're still doing the activity "together" even when you're apart.

3. Write anything you want! You could talk about what's going on in your family, what's happening at school, a funny dream you had, or your dreams for the future—or you could even make up a story. It's up to you.

4. At the end of the week, get together as a family and talk about how the daily journaling felt. Did you like it? Why or why not? Did you learn anything new about yourself or come up with any interesting ideas?

TIPS FOR PARENTS AND CAREGIVERS

Journaling is a well-documented method to help people deal with and learn from big emotions and past challenges. The added benefit of doing this daily journaling challenge as a family is an extra sense of togetherness and belonging.

For your kids who aren't writing letters, encourage them to draw or doodle. It doesn't really matter *what* they put down on the pages; the point is to help your kids learn that they deserve a space to be creative and jot down whatever comes to mind.

Do you think you can always tell how someone else feels?

Maybe someone *looks* angry, sad, or mad—but if you asked them how they're feeling, they might tell you they feel fine or they're just busy concentrating on something, like a tough homework problem. Sometimes the way you *think* someone feels might not actually match what they are truly feeling inside. The only way to know for sure: ask!

Jenga is a fun game of problem-solving, risk, and strategy. This version of Jenga is also a fun way to start a conversation with your family members about your unique feelings and thoughts.

MATERIALS NEEDED	
A Jenga game (same as the one used in activity 15 on page 36)	Permanent markers Sticky notes

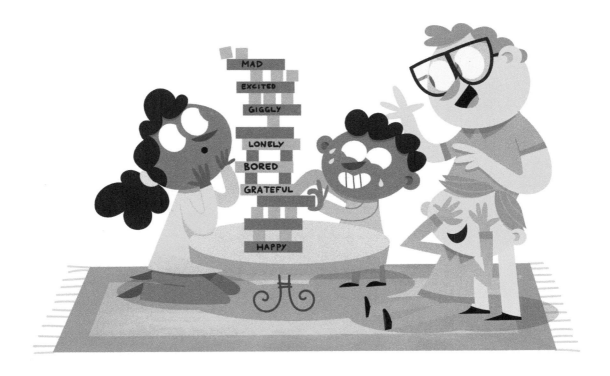

HOW TO DO THE ACTIVITY

1. Get together as a family and spread out your Jenga pieces. Write down a different emotion or feeling on each piece (or as many pieces as you can). Or write the emotions on sitcky notes and stick them to the blocks. If you did activity 15 on page 36, you can reuse the same set of blocks.

2. Stack up your Jenga pieces into a tower, according to the game's directions. There should be three wooden pieces per row, and each row goes in an alternate direction. Ask a grown-up if you need help.

3. Have each family member take turns pulling out a Jenga piece. If a word is written on their Jenga piece, that person should stop and think about a time when they saw someone else in the group show that emotion. For example, a person might pull out a Jenga piece that says "Sad." The person might turn to their stepparent and say, "Last night when you got home from work, I thought you looked really sad." The stepparent can then respond to this by saying how they remember feeling in that moment and why they felt that way.

Keep in mind that this person might agree or disagree about the word on the Jenga piece describing their feeling.

When the Jenga tower finally falls, gather up the wooden blocks, and play again if you wish.

TIPS FOR PARENTS AND CAREGIVERS

Let's face it: Most of us occasionally struggle with identifying exactly how *we* feel, let alone how *other* people feel! Plus, it can be frustrating to have your feelings misinterpreted, even if by accident.

This activity gives everyone in your family a chance to clarify how they feel, and it teaches them that how they feel isn't always "obvious" to others. Guide this activity along by asking prompting questions, such as "Is that how you really felt?" or "Why do you think you felt that way?" or "Can you tell us more about that?"

When you notice that someone close to you isn't feeling their best, what should you do? It really depends on the situation, of course, but a good place to start is to offer some kind, understanding words.

We call this *empathy*. Empathy is showing that you understand how someone feels and that you care.

It's important to know that you can't control how other people feel. Their feelings are *their* feelings, and they are allowed to have them—just like you're allowed to have yours. But you *can* do kind things that may help someone start to change their perspective and eventually feel better. You never know when something you say might change someone's day for the better!

In this activity, you and your family will create a special way to express how much you care for each other.

MATERIALS NEEDED

Empty jars
Paper
Tape

Drawing utensils, such as colored
pencils, markers, or crayons
Kid-safe scissors

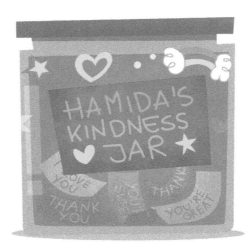

HOW TO DO THE ACTIVITY

1. Sit down as a family. Have each family member make their own kindness jar. Use paper, tape or glue, and other art supplies to label the jars with your names and decorate them how you like.

2. Cut up more paper into long strips that are big enough to write on.

3. Put these kindness jars and strips of paper where everyone can see and reach them, such as on the kitchen counter or a bookshelf.

4. Throughout the week, fill each family member's jar with some kind, thoughtful words. You might want to write down a compliment, something you like or admire about them, words of encouragement, or simply a thank-you for something they do for you regularly.

Here's the rule: anyone can look in their kindness jar whenever they're feeling a bit sad or down. When you look through your jar, notice how your feelings can change when you read all the wonderful, caring things your family members have to say about you.

TIPS FOR PARENTS AND CAREGIVERS

This activity focuses on building empathy—being able to recognize someone else's feelings—and showing your kids that the words they say can have a huge impact on the people around them. As the caregiver, feel free to monitor the jars and ensure that each person's jar is being equally contributed to.

Be sure to provide some positive reinforcement when you notice your kids putting a kind word in a family member's jar; offer a kind word yourself, a hug, or some other act of love. Recognizing when our kids show empathy and rewarding them will help them build this valuable emotional skill.

48 THE KINDNESS PAPER CHAIN

When you're feeling sad, nervous, scared, or some other big emotion, it can be hard to notice all the good things going on around you. But if you stop and look for goodness in this world, I promise that you will find it!

This activity is your chance to sit down with your family and make a "paper chain of kindness." You'll see that kindness *never* runs out, and even if you don't see someone else acting with kindness, you always have the choice to act with kindness at absolutely any moment.

MATERIALS NEEDED

Kid-safe scissors
Paper (construction paper is great for this!)

Pencils or pens
Tape

TIPS FOR PARENTS AND CAREGIVERS

Building on the importance of empathy, this activity helps your kids see how acts of kindness can lead to a "chain" event of kind and loving experiences. That is, when we do something kind for someone else that makes them feel good, that person may want to do something kind for someone else—and on and on it goes.

What I really love about this activity is that your family never really has to be "done" making the chain. Once the initial chain is complete, ask your kids if they can think of *more* kind things they can do. It's wonderful to watch your kids get excited about coming up with creative ways to be kind to each other!

HOW TO DO THE ACTIVITY

1. Use your scissors to cut your paper into long strips that are large enough to write a few words on.

2. Get together as a family and talk about what it means to be kind. How does kindness make us feel? How can we be kind to other people with our thoughts, actions, and words?

3. Take turns thinking about a time when someone was kind to you or when you were kind to someone else. In a few words, write about this moment on one of the strips of paper. Here are some examples:

   - My stepsister let me borrow her favorite toy.

   - I gave my stepdad a hug when he said he felt tired.

   - The mailman gave our dog a dog treat.

   - The school crossing guard has a big smile on her face in the morning.

   - I gave my brother space when he said he wanted to be alone.

4. Once you have a collection of kind memories written on the strips of paper, link them together in a paper chain with tape. Ask your grown-up if you need help!

Watch as your paper chain of kindness grows and grows. There's no limit to how long this chain can get, especially when you work together as a family to start doing more acts of kindness for each other and others!

49 SPEAKER, LISTENER (LET'S TAKE TURNS!)

When you have something to say, it feels good when someone really listens to you. But do you know what it means to be a good listener?

This activity gives you a chance to practice a skill called *active listening*. It's a great way to show someone that you care about them.

MATERIALS NEEDED

Space to sit comfortably with your family

TIPS FOR PARENTS AND CAREGIVERS

It's never too early to start practicing active listening skills. Developing these skills will help your children become effective communicators and make a real impact on the people around them.

It might be helpful to try this role-play activity with each of your children first so you can model what an active listener looks like, offer gentle corrections as needed, and let your kids start to get the hang of what it really means to "put on their listening ears."

HOW TO DO THE ACTIVITY //

1. Pair up with one of your family members. Decide who will be the Speaker and who will be the Listener.

2. The Speaker gets to start talking about something that has been on their mind recently—something they're worried about, something they're struggling with, or any other challenge.

3. The Listener gets to practice active listening. Here are some tips for the Listener:

   • Pay attention. Look at the person as they speak. Keep your own mouth closed and your body still. It might help if you pretend to zip your lips shut or put an imaginary bubble in your mouth.

   • Think about what the other person is saying—don't think about what you want to say yet.

4. When the Speaker has finished talking, it's time for the Listener to ask questions to make sure they understood what the Speaker said. The Listener can ask questions like "What do you mean by that?" or "Tell me about . . ." or "What do you think about . . .?" Give the Speaker a chance to answer these questions.

5. The Listener's next job is to summarize, using their own words, what the Speaker said. (Summarize means to explain the main points of something in a short and simple way.) This shows that the Listener was paying attention and can see things from the Speaker's point of view. At this point, the Listener can also offer their own thoughts, ideas, and suggestions.

6. After you've both shared your thoughts and feelings, switch roles.

When you have something big on your mind, it can feel hard to speak up—and it can also feel hard to speak up when you're interrupted. When someone interrupts you, it's difficult to express yourself fully, and you may forget what you want to say. That's no fun!

In this activity, you and your family will create a tool—the family talking stick—that you can use to help create healthy conversations. A physical object (such as a talking stick) can remind everyone that listening to each other is one of the best ways to show we care.

MATERIALS NEEDED

A stick of any kind: a drumstick, a tree branch, a toilet paper tube—anything!

Arts and crafts materials to decorate your stick

Glue

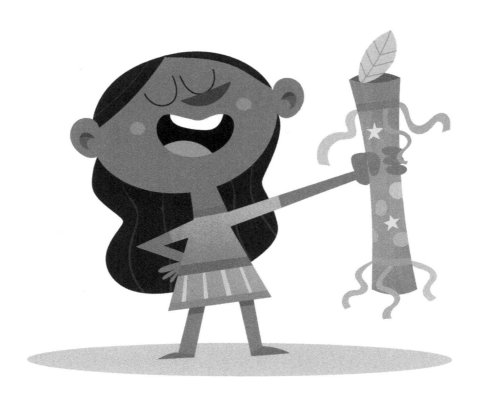

HOW TO DO THE ACTIVITY

1. Gather your drawing utensils.

2. Get together as a family and decorate your talking stick. Be creative!

3. Decide as a family where in your home you want to place this stick.

The rule: Whenever someone is holding the Family Talking Stick, the rest of the family stops and listens—without interrupting. The family talking stick can be passed to other people throughout the conversation so that everyone gets a chance to take turns speaking and listening.

TIPS FOR PARENTS AND CAREGIVERS

Everyone in the family should understand that this talking stick is special and should be used when someone has something big they want to get off their chest. The talking stick should be respected.

If you're concerned that the family talking stick might be used improperly, consider designating specific times to sit together and use it. Also, the talking stick can be used between just two people (such as you and your child) instead of the whole family.

The goal is for your children to associate the sight of this stick with the decision to switch to active listening mode.

YOU DID IT!

Congratulations! You made it!

I'm proud of you and your family for sticking with it and getting involved in some or even all the activities and learning opportunities presented in this book.

By this point, I'm hopeful that you feel:

◆ You've gained some skills that will help you name and really *feel* your feelings—yes, even when they're big!

◆ You've had fun using your creativity and imagination to adjust to your changing family

◆ You've practiced turning your negative feelings into positive ones

◆ You've experienced how fun it is to show yourself and your family members kindness and love—and to try to see things from other people's perspectives

◆ You've started to see how it's possible to learn and grow through new relationships

Most important, I hope you've learned that no matter how your family is changing, *you belong!*

To all the kids out there growing up in a blended family, I want you to know that you have so much to look forward to in life. I truly believe that you have something special to offer your family, your friends, your community, and the world. And in a way, the fact that you've already experienced big feelings and big changes in life is a gift—because it makes you a stronger person.

Remember, even if your parents aren't married anymore, they still love you as much as ever. Even if you get to have a stepparent, nobody can replace either of your parents. And even if you and your siblings now have *new* siblings to get to know, you still have an important role to play in your growing family. You are loved, you are wanted, and you are safe.

To the parents and caregivers, thank you for joining in on this journey. I know that navigating divorce, entering new relationships, and guiding your family as it changes can be challenging. My hope is that the activities in this book have given you and your kids some new tools and ideas for taking good care of yourselves as you go through some major life changes.

Because let's face it: when you take care of *you*, your whole family benefits.

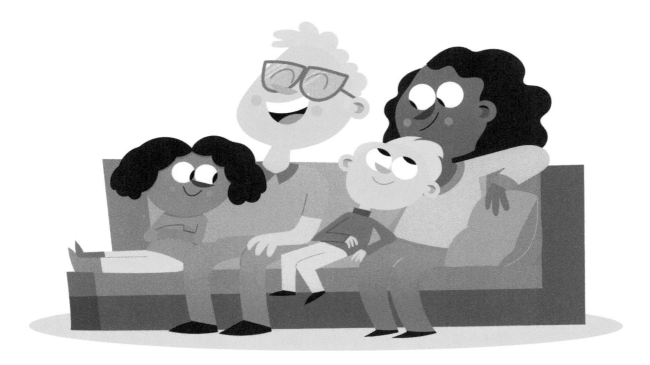

RESOURCES

RESOURCES FOR KIDS

A Family Is a Family Is a Family, Sarah O'Leary
A fun book that invites you to think about all the things that make your family special.

Blended, Sharon M. Draper
Read this book as a family to hear an important perspective about divorce, race, and what it means to be a family.

DivorceCare for Kids
With your parents, check out dc4k.org to connect with other kids who are part of blended families! Discover games, stories, videos, music, and conversations to develop new skills and help yourself heal in a safe and fun environment.

Living with Mom and Living with Dad, Melanie Walsh
This beautiful, interactive book helps you gain a new outlook on living in two homes with two growing families.

Sesame Street in Communities: Dealing with Divorce
Join your favorite Sesame Street characters as you explore resources and activities that will help you understand what being in a blended family means for you.

SPLIT
SPLIT is a short film for kids (and their caregivers) about divorce. Grab some popcorn and watch it here: SplitFilm.org.

The List of Things That Will Not Change, Rebecca Stead
A novel about divorce, forgiving mistakes, and accepting ourselves—even as our families go through major changes.

RESOURCES FOR PARENTS AND CAREGIVERS

***Blending Families*, Jimmy Evans**
Read this book to gain insights from real blended families that will help your own changing family thrive.

***Co-parenting After Divorce: A GPS for Kids*, Debra K. Carter**
In this book, you'll learn helpful tools and strategies, with or without a parenting coordinator, to develop an effective parenting plan that will help your kids navigate the sometimes bumpy road of parental divorce.

Divorce and Children
A comprehensive hub of resources, including articles and personal coaching sessions, for separated and divorced parents: DivorceAndChildren.com.

***Journey Beyond Divorce* Podcast**
Journey Beyond Divorce is the "leading on-line or in-person source for the best divorce coaches to assist you through your difficult transition." The *Journey Beyond Divorce* podcast is hosted by divorce and relationship coach Karen McMahon.

***Our Happy Divorce*, Nikki DeBartolo and Benjamin Heldfond**
This book is available to anyone interested in a new perspective on divorce, coparenting, and stepparenting.

The Divorce Survival Guide Podcast
Recommended by the *New York Times*, *The Divorce Survival Guide Podcast* is hosted by certified divorce coach Kate Anthony. You can also download her *Ultimate Divorce Survival Guide* here: KateAnthony.com/getting-divorced.

REFERENCES

Chapman, Gary. *The 5 Love Languages*. Chicago: Northfield Publishing, 1992.

Harvard Heath Publishing. "Writing about Emotions May Ease Stress and Trauma." Harvard Medical School. October 11, 2011. Health.Harvard.edu/healthbeat /writing-about-emotions-may-ease-stress-and-trauma.

Viorst, Judith. *Alexander and the Terrible, Horrible, No Good, Very Bad Day*. New York: Atheneum Books for Young Readers, 1972.

INDEX

ABOUT THE AUTHOR

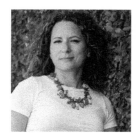

April Eldemire, LMFT, is a nationally recognized licensed marriage and family therapist from Fort Lauderdale, Florida. She earned her bachelor's degree in psychology from Florida State University in 2004, followed by her master's degree in marriage and family therapy along with a minor in conflict analysis and resolution from Nova Southeastern University in 2007.

In addition to running her own private counseling practice, April is a guest blogger and regular contributor for the Gottman Institute. She has been featured as a marriage expert in the *Boca Raton Observer* and *Brides* magazines and has been interviewed on the *Mastering Counseling* podcast.

In her free time, she loves hanging out with her family, staying active, and cooking healthy meals for her family.

ABOUT THE ILLUSTRATOR

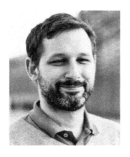

Amir Abou-Roumié is an illustrator with a focus on children's and humorous illustrations with over 10 years of experience based in Vienna, Austria. He has illustrated and animated for exhibitions, websites, school books, advertising campaigns, pharmaceutical products, mobile applications, and educational projects for kids. His illustrations are inspired by the reduced cartoon and animation art of the 40s, 50s and 60s, but also influenced by contemporary works. You can find him at AmirAbouRoumie.com

CPSIA information can be obtained
at www.ICGtesting.com
Printed in the USA
BVHW020750200122
626692BV00005B/10